CALCULATIONS FOR
VETERINARY NURSES

Dedication

The authors would like to dedicate this book to
Vic Moore
in appreciation of all his
hard work as our 'unofficial' editor and advisor

Acknowledgements

The authors would like to thank their spouses
Vic Moore and Sylvia Palmer
for their patience and understanding
during the time taken to write this book

CALCULATIONS FOR VETERINARY NURSES

Margaret C. Moore
MA, VN, Cert Ed, FETC. MIScT

and

Norman G. Palmer

Blackwell
Science

© 2001 by
Blackwell Science Ltd
Editorial Offices:
Osney Mead, Oxford OX2 0EL
25 John Street, London WC1N 2BS
23 Ainslie Place, Edinburgh EN3 6AJ
350 Main Street, Malden
  MA 02148 5018, USA
54 University Street, Carlton
  Victoria 3053, Australia
10, rue Casimir Delavigne
  75006 Paris, France

Other Editorial Offices

Blackwell Wissenschafts-Verlag GmbH
Kurfürstendamm 57
10707 Berlin, Germany

Blackwell Science KK
MG Kodenmacho Building
7–10 Kodenmacho Nihombashi
Chuo-ku, Tokyo 104, Japan

Iowa State University Press
A Blackwell Science Company
2121 S. State Avenue
Ames, Iowa 50014–8300, USA

The right of the Author to be identified as
the Author of this Work has been asserted
in accordance with the Copyright, Designs
and Patents Act 1988.

First published 2001

Set in Souvenir 9/11½ pt
by Aarontype, Easton, Bristol
Printed and bound in Great Britain by
MPG Books, Bodmin, Cornwall

The Blackwell Science logo is a
trade mark of Blackwell Science Ltd,
registered at the United Kingdom
Trade marks Regisrty

DISTRIBUTORS
Marston Book Services Ltd
PO Box 269
Abingdon
Oxon OX14 4YN
(Orders: Tel: 01235 465500
        Fax: 01235 465555)

USA and Canada
Iowa State University Press
A Blackwell Science Company
2121 S. State Avenue
Ames, Iowa 50014–8300
(Orders: Tel: 800–862–6657
        Fax: 515–292–3348
        Web: www.isupress.com
        email: orders@isupress.com)

Australia
Blackwell Science Pty Ltd
54 University Street
Carlton, Victoria 3053
(Orders: Tel: 03 9347 0300
        Fax: 03 9347 5001)

A catalogue record for this title
is available from the British Library

ISBN 0–632–05498–0

Library of Congress
Cataloging-in-Publication Data

Moore Margaret C., M.A.
  Calculations for veterinary
  nurses / Margaret C. Moore and
  Norman G. Palmer.
    p. cm.
  ISBN 0–632–05498–0 (pbk.)
  1. Veterinary drugs – Dosage.
  I. Palmer, Norman G. II. Title

  SF919 .M66 2000
  636.089'514—dc21

                              00–046797

For further information on
Blackwell Science, visit our website:
www.blackwell-science.com

Contents

Preface

Currently, there are excellent technical books available for both student and qualified veterinary nurses. However, no single publication encompasses all the different types of calculations on which student veterinary nurses may be examined or which qualified veterinary nurses are expected to carry out routinely during the course of their work.

During twenty years as a course tutor for veterinary nurses, my own students have repeatedly indicated the need for such a book. Thus the aim of this volume is to meet that need by including a separate section on each of the different calculations which a veterinary nurse is likely to use.

It is structured in such a way that the reader can progress from a simple explanation of the principles involved to their application of essential veterinary calculations.

Numerous worked examples are included together with self-test exercises which, where appropriate, have also been supported with fully-worked answers. The aim of this approach is to help readers understand the arithmetic principles needed to perform basic calculations, thus enabling them to have the confidence and ability to carry out any veterinary calculations which they are likely to come across during the course of their careers.

Although this book is designed primarily to assist student veterinary nurses for whom calculations are an essential part of their studies, it will undoubtedly be an invaluable aide-mémoire and reference for qualified staff. It will also be an extremely valuable text book for students following other animal-based careers, for example, animal technicians and animal carers. In discussing this book with veterinary surgeons, many of them kindly expressed the view that it may also be of use to veterinary students.

Disclaimer

The primary aim of this book is to explain how to carry out basic veterinary calculations. To achieve this, some of the figures used have given way to convenience of calculation rather than adhering to clinical accuracy. Finally, any similarities to animals, whether living or dead, are purely coincidental!

Note

All answers to worked examples appear in bold type.

Margaret C. Moore
Norman G. Palmer

Common Abbreviations Used in Text

Weight

g   gram(s)
kg   kilogram(s)
mg   milligram(s)
mcg   microgram(s)

Volume

ℓ   litre(s)
ml   millilitre(s)

Time

min   minute(s)
s   second(s)
hr(s)   hour(s)

Unit·of electric current

mA   milliampere(s)

Unit of electromotive force

kV   kilovolt

Chapter 1

Units, Conversion Factors and Related Medical Abbreviations

It is imperative that a good understanding of units and the relationship between them is gained at an early stage when studying calculations. Many of the problems encountered whilst carrying out basic calculations stem from a lack of understanding of the units in which various quantities are measured, and of the relationships between them. A thorough working knowledge of the most common units is vital to anyone in the veterinary nursing profession. A mistake in the use of units could be fatal to a patient.

The metric system of weights and measures is now used by the veterinary profession in most countries. It is international and simpler to use than any other system. Thus it is the safest to use because mistakes are less likely to occur. The units which are most commonly used in the veterinary profession are shown below.

Weight

1 kilogram (kg)	= 1000 grams (1000 g)
1 gram (g)	= 1000 milligrams (1000 mg)
1 milligram (mg)	= 1000 micrograms
	(1000 μg also referred to as mcg)
1 microgram (μg)	= 1000 nanograms (1000 ng)

Length

    1 kilometre (km) = 1000 metres (1000 m)
    1 metre (m)   = 100 centimetres (100 cm)
    1 centimetre (cm) = 10 millimetres (10 mm)

Volume

    1 litre (ℓ)   = 1000 millilitres (1000 ml)
    1 decilitre (dl) = 100 millilitres (100 ml)

Notes

- Centimetres are not used as frequently as millimetres and metres. Therefore instead of a certain length being described as 10 cm, it is more likely to be referred to as 100 mm or 0.1 m.
- 1 gram of water occupies 1 millilitre of space (at 15°C). Therefore, 1000 ml or 1 litre of water will weigh 1000 grams or 1 kilogram.
- To help avoid confusion weights of less than 1 gram should be written as milligrams e.g. 500 mg rather than 0.5 g. Similarly, weights of less than 1 milligram should be written in micrograms.
- The letter 'L' in upper case is sometimes used as an abbreviation for litre. See note after examples below.
- mcg is sometimes used in pharmacy as an abbreviation for micrograms.

Abbreviations and prefixes

The abbreviation for each of the common units is normally the first letter of the name. Thus the abbreviation for metre is m and the abbreviation for gram is g. In order to express a multiple of a unit, prefixes are placed in front of the name. The common prefixes are shown in table 1.1.

Table 1.1 Common prefixes

Prefix	Symbol	Value	Multiplies by
deci	d	0.1	one tenth
centi	c	0.01	one hundredth
milli	m	0.001	one thousandth
micro	μ	0.000001	one millionth
deca	da	10	ten
kilo	k	1000	one thousand
mega	M	1 000 000	one million

Notes

- When a prefix is used with a unit of measurement, the abbreviation for the prefix is followed by the abbreviation for the unit, e.g. 25 millilitres is written as 25 ml.
- Although 25 ml obviously refers to the plural of the word millilitre, there is no letter 's' added, i.e. 25 millilitres is *not* written as 25 mls. This rule applies to all of the units listed above.

Examples

Write the abbreviations for the units together with the appropriate prefix when necessary for the following:

(i) Twenty one millilitres
     Answer: 21 ml

(ii) Twenty one litres
     Answer: 21 ℓ or 21 L (*see note below*)

(iii) Twenty one milligrams
     Answer: 21 mg

(iv) Twenty one micrograms
     Answer: 21 µg

Note

The abbreviation for litre is the letter 'l' in lower case but this abbreviation could cause confusion when it is preceded by the digit one, i.e. 21 l could be mistaken for the figure 211. In order to avoid the possibility of such a mistake, the abbreviation for the litre is sometimes written as 'L' so that in the above example, twenty one litres would be written as 21 L. In this book, the symbol ℓ is used to denote litres.

Converting units within the metric system

The most frequent conversions used in the veterinary profession are likely to involve volumes and weights.

Examples

Convert the following:

(i) 750 g to kg

There are 1000 grams in 1 kilogram, therefore to convert grams to kilograms, divide by 1000 (move the decimal point 3 places to the left). For a full explanation see Chapter 2.

$$\text{Therefore } 750\,g = \frac{750}{1000}\,kg = \textbf{0.750\,kg}$$

(ii) 7.50 g to kg

There are 1000 grams in 1 kilogram, therefore to convert grams to kilograms, divide by 1000 (move the decimal point 3 places to the left).

Therefore $7.50\,\text{g} = \dfrac{7.50}{1000}\,\text{kg} = \mathbf{0.0075\,kg}$

(iii)   750 mg to g

There are 1000 milligrams in 1 gram therefore to convert milligrams to grams, divide by 1000 (move the decimal point 3 places to the left).

Therefore $750\,\text{mg} = \dfrac{750}{1000}\,\text{g} = \mathbf{0.750\,g}$

(iv)   750 μg to g

There are 1 000 000 (one million) micrograms in 1 gram, therefore to convert micrograms to grams, divide by 1 000 000 (move the decimal point 6 places to the left).

Therefore $750\,\mu\text{g} = \dfrac{750}{1\,000\,000}\,\text{g} = \mathbf{0.000750\,g}$

(v)   0.0075 g to mg

There are 1000 milligrams in 1 gram, therefore to convert grams to milligrams, multiply by 1000 (move the decimal point 3 places to the right).

Therefore $0.0075\,\text{g} = 0.0075 \times 1000\,\text{mg} = \mathbf{7.5\,mg}$

(vi)   0.750 mg to μg

There are 1000 micrograms in 1 milligram, therefore to convert milligrams to micrograms, multiply by 1000 (move the decimal point 3 places to the right).

Therefore $0.750\,\text{mg} = 0.750 \times 1000\,\mu\text{g} = \mathbf{750\,\mu g}$

(vii)   750 ml to litres

There are 1000 millilitres in 1 litre, therefore to convert millilitres to litres, divide by 1000 (move the decimal point 3 places to the left).

Therefore $750 \, \text{ml} = \dfrac{750}{1000} \, \ell = \mathbf{0.750 \, \ell}$

(viii) $7.50 \, \ell$ to ml

There are 1000 millilitres in 1 litre, therefore to convert litres to millilitres, multiply by 1000 (move the decimal point 3 places to the right).

Therefore $7.50 \, \ell = 7.50 \times 1000 \, \text{ml} = \mathbf{7500 \, ml}$

(ix) $0.0750 \, \ell$ to ml

There are 1000 millilitres in 1 litre, therefore to convert litres to millilitres, multiply by 1000 (move the decimal point 3 places to the right).

Therefore $0.0750 \, \ell = 0.0750 \times 1000 \, \text{ml} = \mathbf{75.0 \, ml}$

Converting 'old' imperial units to metric values

The imperial system of units is being phased out. However, some of the 'everyday' units are likely to remain in use for many years and it is therefore important to be able to understand the abbreviations used and to be able to convert the units to their metric equivalents.

The most common conversions used by the veterinary profession are shown in table 1.2.

Table 1.2 Common conversion factors

Imperial unit	To convert multiply by	Metric
lb	0.45	kg
pt (pint)	0.57	ℓ (litres)
in (inch)	25.4	mm
fl oz (fluid ounce)	28.4	ml

Examples

Convert the following imperial units into their metric equivalents.

(i)   20 lb

  To convert lb to kg multiply by 0.45
  Therefore 20 lb = 20 × 0.45 kg = **9 kg**

(ii)   10 lb

  To convert lb to kg multiply by 0.45
  Therefore 10 lb = 10 × 0.45 kg = **4.5 kg**

Note to multiply by 10, move the decimal point one place to the right.

(iii)   0.5 lb

  To convert lb to kg multiply by 0.45
  Therefore 0.5 lb = 0.5 × 0.45 kg = **0.225 kg**

(iv)   1.5 pt

  To convert pt to ℓ multiply by 0.57
  Therefore 1.5 pt = 1.5 × 0.57 ℓ = **0.86 ℓ** (to 2 decimal places)

(v)   30 in

  To convert in to mm multiply by 25.4
  Therefore 30 in = 30 × 25.4 mm = **762 mm**

(vi)   3 fl oz

  To convert fl oz to ml multiply by 28.4
  Therefore 3 fl oz = 3 × 28.4 ml = **85.2ml**

'Household' or 'domestic' measurement system

Several units of measurement are based on the volumes of common household utensils. These units are still widely used by

Table 1.3 Approximate volume of 'household' measurements

Household measurement	Approximate volume in ml
Standard teaspoon	5
Standard dessert spoon	10
Standard table spoon	15
Teacup	150
Twelve drops	5

manufacturers of such products as disinfectants or animal shampoos, which may be sold via pet shops etc. to people who do not have access to accurate volumetric measuring equipment or who are not familiar with the metric system of units. The 'household' units are also invaluable when giving advice to, or eliciting information from, clients over the telephone. For instance, when describing clinical signs, a client may state that 'my dog has vomited and produced about a teaspoon of bile'.

It is because of the practical application of these units that a knowledge of their metric equivalents is occasionally tested in the RCVS Veterinary Nursing examinations. The most commonly used of the 'household' units are shown in table 1.3.

Note

Under no circumstances should these conversions be used for measuring out drugs.

Temperature conversions

An examination of the Celsius and Fahrenheit scales will reveal that each degree on the Celsius scale is nearly twice as big as a Fahrenheit degree. This is because on the Celsius scale there are only 100 degrees between the freezing and boiling points (of water), whilst on the Fahrenheit scale there are 212 degrees between the freezing and boiling points. A further obvious difference is that the freezing point on the Celsius scale is zero, whilst on the Fahrenheit scale it is 32. These differences are the reason that temperature conversions have to be carried out in stages using one of the methods shown below.

Notes

- The correct name of the temperature unit is Celsius not Centigrade.
- Method 2 below is based on the fact that $-40\,^{\circ}$C is the same as $-40\,^{\circ}$F

To convert from Fahrenheit to Celsius

Method 1

- First subtract 32 (This takes account of the difference in freezing points)
- Next multiply by $\frac{5}{9}$ (This takes account of the size difference)

Method 2

- First add 40
- Next multiply by $\frac{5}{9}$
- Finally subtract 40

To convert from Celsius to Fahrenheit

Method 1

- First multiply by $\frac{9}{5}$
- Next add 32

Method 2

- First add 40
- Next multiply by $\frac{9}{5}$
- Finally subtract 40

Examples

Convert the following temperatures from Fahrenheit to Celsius.

(i)   A room temperature of 50°F

Method 1

$50 - 32 = 18$
$18 \times \frac{5}{9} = \mathbf{10}°\mathbf{C}$

Method 2

$50 + 40 = 90$
$90 \times \frac{5}{9} = 50$
$50 - 40 = \mathbf{10}°\mathbf{C}$

(ii)   A guinea pig's temperature of 104°F

Method 1

$104 - 32 = 72$
$72 \times \frac{5}{9} = \mathbf{40}°\mathbf{C}$

Method 2

$104 + 40 = 144$
$144 \times \frac{5}{9} = 80$
$80 - 40 = \mathbf{40}°\mathbf{C}$

(iii)   A chinchilla's temperature of 97°F

Method 1

$97 - 32 = 65$
$65 \times \frac{5}{9} = \mathbf{36.1}°\mathbf{C}$

Method 2

$97 + 40 = 137$
$137 \times \frac{5}{9} = 76.1$
$76.1 - 40 = \mathbf{36.1}°\mathbf{C}$

Convert the following temperatures from Celsius to Fahrenheit.

(i)   A hamster's temperature of 37°C

Method 1

$37 \times \frac{9}{5} = 66.6$
$66.6 + 32 = \mathbf{98.6}°\mathbf{F}$

Method 2

$37 + 40 = 77$
$77 \times \frac{9}{5} = 138.6$
$138.6 - 40 = \mathbf{98.6}°\mathbf{F}$

(ii)   An autoclave temperature of 120°C

Method 1

$120 \times \frac{9}{5} = 216$
$216 + 32 = \mathbf{248}°\mathbf{F}$

Method 2

$120 + 40 = 160$
$160 \times \frac{9}{5} = 288$
$288 - 40 = \mathbf{248}°\mathbf{F}$

Related medical abbreviations

u.i.d.	once daily
u.d.s.	to be taken once daily
o.d.	every day (used to mean once a day)
b.i.d or b.d.	twice daily
b.d.s.	to be taken twice daily
t.i.d. or t.d.	3 times a day
t.d.s.	to be taken 3 times a day
q.i.d. or q.d.	4 times a day
q.d.s.	to be taken 4 times a day
q.h.	every 4 hours
altern.d	every other day
p.r.n.	repeat as required
repet. or rep.	repeat
a.c.	before food
p.c.	after food
o.m.	every morning
o.n.	every night

Chapter 2

Basic Principles

In order to carry out veterinary calculations, it is necessary to have a working knowledge of a few simple but essential arithmetic concepts. This chapter explains how to perform these basic calculations. The method of carrying out each type of calculation is illustrated with worked examples and self-test exercises.

Fractions

A fraction is another word for a part of something; for instance, a tablet could be broken into two equal sized parts, i.e. 1 divided by 2 which is written as $\frac{1}{2}$. In this case, each part or fraction is called a half. If the tablet was broken into four equal sized parts, i.e. 1 divided by 4, then each part or fraction would be called a quarter and written as $\frac{1}{4}$.

The above examples may seem fairly obvious but the situation may arise where something has to be divided into many more parts. For instance, an hour is divided into 60 equal fractions called minutes or, put another way, a minute is one sixtieth ($\frac{1}{60}$) of an hour.

Further complications arise when something is broken into uneven parts; for instance, a can of food may be divided between three dogs in such a way that one of them receives twice as much as the other two. In this case, the can of food will be divided into one half and two quarters which, added together, would equal one whole can or, putting this in mathematical terms, $\frac{1}{4} + \frac{1}{4} + \frac{1}{2} = 1$.

The number on the top line of a fraction is known as the *numerator* and the one on the bottom line is the *denominator*. It should be noted that the larger the denominator in relation to the numerator, the smaller each part or fraction will be. For instance the fraction $\frac{1}{6}$ will be smaller than the fraction $\frac{1}{3}$.

Similarly, $\frac{3}{10}$ is smaller than $\frac{3}{7}$ and so on. It should also be noted that some calculations produce rather complicated looking fractions, e.g. $\frac{350}{400}$. Sometimes fractions are produced in which the numerator is larger than the denominator, e.g. $\frac{16}{12}$. These are known as improper fractions, as opposed to proper fractions, in which the numerator is smaller than the denominator.

Simplifying fractions (cancelling)

Complicated fractions are confusing to use in calculations and even more difficult to translate into practical applications; for instance, how can $\frac{12}{60}$ of a bag of dog food be measured out? What does such a fraction mean in everyday terms? In order to deal with complicated fractions, they have to be cancelled or simplified.

Cancelling a fraction is the process of dividing both the top and bottom lines by the *same number* in order to produce a simpler (and more understandable) fraction.

Example 1

The fraction $\frac{14}{28}$ can be cancelled by dividing both the top and the bottom by 7.
This produces $\frac{2}{4}$ which can be cancelled further by dividing both the top and bottom by 2.
This produces $\frac{1}{2}$.
The above cancelling process has actually shown that
14 divided by 28 $= \frac{1}{2}$.

Example 2

The fraction $\frac{21}{63}$ can be cancelled by dividing both the top and the bottom by 7.

This produces $\frac{3}{9}$ which can be cancelled further by dividing both the top and bottom by 3.

This produces $\frac{1}{3}$ which cannot be cancelled or simplified any further.

Example 3

Returning to the problem mentioned above which involved measuring out $\frac{12}{60}$ of a bag of dog food, it can be seen that the top and bottom of the fraction can both be divided by 12. This will produce a much simpler fraction of $\frac{1}{5}$ which indicates more clearly that the bag will have to be divided into 5 equal portions.

Example 4

The fraction $\frac{300}{12\,000}$ looks quite complicated at first sight but because both the numerator and the denominator end in zeros, it can be simplified very quickly by cancelling out the zeros. In this case, two of the zeros on the top will cancel out two of the zeros on the bottom. In other words, both the top and the bottom can be divided by 100.

This produces $\frac{3}{120}$ which can be cancelled further by dividing both the top and bottom by 3.

This produces $\frac{1}{40}$.

Self-test exercise 1
(answers at the end of this chapter)

Simplify the following fractions.

(i) $\frac{25}{5}$ (ii) $\frac{34}{68}$ (iii) $\frac{57}{19}$ (iv) $\frac{27}{36}$ (v) $\frac{31}{93}$

(vi) $\frac{18}{4}$ (vii) $\frac{3}{6}$ (viii) $\frac{20}{15}$ (ix) $\frac{54}{18}$ (x) $\frac{112}{4}$

Converting fractions to decimals

It is possible to add, subtract, multiply and divide fractions but the easiest way to perform these tasks is to convert the fractions into their decimal equivalents first. To convert a fraction to its decimal equivalent, divide the numerator by the denominator. It is suggested that a calculator is used for this purpose.

Example 1

$\frac{3}{10}$ expressed as a decimal $= \mathbf{0.3}$

Note that when a decimal value is less than one it will begin with the decimal point. In such cases a zero should be placed to the left of the decimal point in order to prevent confusion. In this case, the zero helps to clarify that the value is 0.3 and not 3.0.

Example 2

$\frac{7}{5}$ expressed as a decimal $= \mathbf{1.4}$

Self-test exercise 2
(answers at the end of this chapter)

Change the following fractions into decimals:

(i) $\frac{25}{50}$ (ii) $\frac{34}{68}$ (iii) $\frac{57}{90}$ (iv) $\frac{29}{87}$ (v) $\frac{31}{17}$

(vi) $\frac{18}{24}$ (vii) $\frac{3}{5}$ (viii) $\frac{20}{45}$ (ix) $\frac{54}{68}$ (x) $\frac{112}{345}$

Rounding decimals

Decimal calculations often produce answers with many digits after the decimal point. Sometimes these digits appear to (and in fact some do) go on forever. An instance of such a figure would be the result of converting the fraction $\frac{2}{3}$ into a decimal. Dividing 2 by 3 produces an answer of 0.666666666 ... Similarly, dividing 30 by 7 produces an answer of 4.2857142. The use of such extremely accurate figures for dispensing solids or liquids in everyday life is normally neither necessary nor practical. Therefore, decimal numbers are rounded to give the appropriate degree of accuracy. To round a decimal number, first determine how accurate the final figure must be; for example, when recording the temperature of an animal, an accuracy of $\frac{1}{10}$ (one tenth) of a degree (0.1) is sufficient. This is known as an accuracy of one decimal place. Some injectables require a syringe marked in graduations of $\frac{1}{100}$ (one hundredth) of a ml (0.01). This is known as an accuracy of two decimal places. Once the required accuracy has been determined, the decimal figure can be rounded accordingly. The basic principle of rounding is to examine the digit to the *right* of the number of decimal places required. When this digit is 5 or greater, it is rounded up i.e. it is removed but the digit to *its immediate left* is increased by 1. When the digit to the *right* of the number of decimal places required is less than 5, it is removed but this time no change is made to the digit to its immediate left.

Example 1

To round 2.36 to one decimal place (or the nearest tenth), the digit 6 will be removed but because it is greater than 5 the digit located to its immediate left will be increased by 1.

Thus the rounded figure $= \mathbf{2.4}$

Example 2

To round 2.34 to one decimal place (or the nearest tenth), the digit 4 will be removed but because it is not greater than 5, the digit located to its immediate left will not be increased by 1.

Thus the rounded figure $= \mathbf{2.3}$

Example 3

To round 2.457 to two decimal places (or the nearest hundredth), the digit 7 will be removed but because it is greater than 5, the digit located to its immediate left will be increased by 1.

Thus the rounded figure = **2.46**

Example 4

To round 2.5 to the nearest whole number, the digit 5 will be removed but because it is 5 or greater, the digit located to its immediate left will be increased by 1.

Thus the rounded figure = **3**

Example 5

To round 2.4 to the nearest whole number, the digit 4 will be removed but because it is less than 5 the digit located to its immediate left will not be increased by 1.

Thus the rounded figure = **2**

Self-test exercise 3
(answers at the end of this chapter)

Round the following figures to the nearest whole number

(i)   9.88   (ii)   9.088   (iii)   9.0088

Round the following figures to one decimal place (nearest tenth)

(iv)   9.88   (v)   9.088   (vi)   9.0088

Round the following figures to two decimal places (nearest hundredth)

(vii)   9.88   (viii)   9.088   (ix)   9.0088

Moving the decimal point

Any whole number can be easily multiplied by 10, 100, 1000 etc. by adding

one zero for 10
two zeros for 100
three zeros for 1000, and so on.

For instance, the number 99.0 becomes 990.0 when multiplied by 10. Similarly, any whole number can be easily divided by 10, 100, 1000 etc. by removing

one zero for 10
two zeros for 100
three zeros for 1000, and so on.

Therefore, 9900 becomes 99 when divided by 100. However, dividing numbers which do not end in a zero involves moving the decimal point. This procedure is explained below.

Decimal numbers can be very easily multiplied or divided by 10, 100, 1000 etc. The golden rule is to move the decimal point

one place for 10
two places for 100
three places for 1000, and so on.

When *dividing* the decimal point is moved to the left. When *multiplying* it is moved to the right. When necessary, additional zeros may have to be added as shown in examples (iii) and (vi) which follow.

Examples

(i)   The number 99.99 becomes 999.9 when multiplied by 10
(ii) The number 99.99 becomes 9999.0 when multiplied by 100
(iii) The number 99.99 becomes 99990.0 when multiplied by 1000
(iv) The number 99.99 becomes 9.999 when divided by 10
(v)   The number 99.99 becomes 0.9999 when divided by 100
(vi) The number 99.99 becomes 0.09999 when divided by 1000

The above principles can be easily proved by using a calculator!

Notes

- A decimal point has been inserted after the whole numbers to avoid confusion. It would not normally be shown, i.e. the number 9999 would be written as such and not 9999.0
- A zero is often placed at the end of a decimal figure to indicate that there are no more digits to follow.

Self-test exercise 4 (answers at the end of this chapter)

(i) Multiply the following figures by 10
50, 5, 0.5, 0.05

(ii) Multiply the following figures by 100
50, 5, 0.5, 0.05

(iii) Multiply the following figures by 1000
50, 5, 0.5, 0.05

(iv) Divide the following figures by 10
6000, 6, 0.6, 0.06

(v) Divide the following figures by 100
6000, 6, 0.6, 0.06

(vi) Divide the following figures by 1000
6000, 6, 0.6, 0.06

Converting fractions into percentages

To convert a fraction to a percentage, first convert to its decimal equivalent by dividing the numerator by the denominator. Then multiply the answer by 100. Note that it is sometimes possible to simplify the fraction at the same time!

Example 1

$\frac{3}{10}$ expressed as a percentage $= \frac{3}{10} \times 100 = \frac{300}{10} = \frac{30}{1} = \mathbf{30\%}$

Example 2

$\frac{10}{3}$ expressed as a percentage $= \dfrac{10}{3} \times 100 = \dfrac{1000}{300} = \mathbf{333.33\%}$

Self-test exercise 5
(answers at the end of this chapter)

Convert the following fractions into percentages:

(i) $\frac{25}{50}$ (ii) $\frac{34}{68}$ (iii) $\frac{57}{36}$ (iv) $\frac{27}{36}$ (v) $\frac{31}{17}$

(vi) $\frac{18}{24}$ (vii) $\frac{3}{13}$ (viii) $\frac{20}{60}$ (ix) $\frac{54}{117}$ (x) $\frac{112}{293}$

Percentages

Percentage is another way of saying 'how many out of 100'. For example, if 20 sheep in a flock of 100 are black, then the percentage of black sheep is 20%. Any percentage can be represented as a fraction of 100, therefore 20% can be expressed as $\frac{20}{100}$. In this case the fraction could be simplified (or cancelled) by dividing both the top and bottom by 20 to produce $\frac{1}{5}$. In other words, expressing the situation as a fraction, it could be stated that one fifth of the sheep are black. Percentages are also easily converted into their decimal equivalents by dividing the number by 100 or by moving the decimal point two places to the left as previously explained.

Percentages appear in almost all areas of everyday and professional life. In an everyday situation they will appear, for example, in relation to interest rates in banks and building societies.

Professionally, veterinary staff will encounter them being used to express

- the amount of solute in a solution expressed as a percentage solution of the amount of concentrate in 100 ml of fluid.
- the number of different types of white cells when compared to the total of white cells expressed as a percentage (differential white blood cell counts).

As 'per-cent-age' means 'how many per one hundred', the use of percentages provides a way to compare varying samples, with different constituent parts on a common base.

For example, the results of a differential white blood (leucocyte) count are likely to show the following leucocyte types (basophils are not included here as they are very rare and are therefore unlikely to be recorded in a typical blood profile). For the purpose of these examples, the different leucocyte types will be given type numbers.

Type 1   Unlobulated (band) neutrophils
Type 2   Lobulated (adult) neutrophils
Type 3   Eosinophils
Type 4   Lymphocytes
Type 5   Monocytes

The amount of each type of leucocyte is recorded and then a simple calculation made e.g. white blood cell (leucocyte) count as shown in table 2.1:

Table 2.1 Differential leucocyte count

Batch No.	Type 1	Type 2	Type 3	Type 4	Type 5	Total cell count
No.1	60	70	14	16	40	200
Type %	30%	35%	7%	8%	20%	100%

Example 1

Type 1: 60 cells counted out of the total 200 leucocytes counted.

Therefore, to find the percentage: $\dfrac{60}{200} \times 100 = \textbf{30\%}$

Type 2: 70 cells counted out of the total 200 leucocytes counted.

Therefore, to find the percentage: $\dfrac{70}{200} \times 100 = \textbf{35\%}$

These calculations may be continued for the whole of batch no. 1. When possible, it is good practice to try and count 200 leucocytes in a differential white blood cell count to increase the range of cells encountered, or a minimum of 100 leucocytes if the cells are difficult to find. Working with total figures of 200 or 100 makes the conversion of the individual types into percentages easy, and once accustomed to the calculation, the results can be converted at a glance.

However, if the animal has leucopenia (a decrease in the total number of leucocytes), then it may be impossible to find such amounts and the total number of leucocytes that can be seen once the whole slide has been searched may be very low. It is still necessary to convert such results into percentages for a differential white cell count.

Example 2

Which of these three solutions is the most concentrated?

Solution A has 25 g of solute dissolved in 750 ml of solution
Solution B has 253 g of solute dissolved in 1750 ml of solution
Solution C has 2.56 g of solute dissolved in 78 ml of solution

Just by looking at these figures it would be impossible to tell which was the most concentrated. Reduce them all to percentages and the answer will stand out immediately!

Solution A $\quad \dfrac{25}{750} \times 100 = \mathbf{3.33\%}$

Solution B $\quad \dfrac{253}{1750} \times 100 = \mathbf{14.46\%}$

Solution C $\quad \dfrac{2.56}{78} \times 100 = \mathbf{3.28\%}$

Obviously solution B is the most concentrated but A and C have similar concentrations, although the basic data vary considerably. From these examples it can be seen that the use of percentages is a powerful comparison tool.

Example 3

Which of the following solutions contains the most solute by weight?

(i)   Solution y: 750 ml of a 5% solution
(ii) Solution x: 1200 ml of a 2% solution
(iii) Solution z: 800 ml of a 4% solution

Calculation: (see manipulating formulae (equations) later in this chapter)

$$\% \text{ solution} = \frac{\textbf{weight in g}}{\textbf{volume in ml}} \times \textbf{100}$$

To rearrange the equation, first multiply both sides by volume.

$$\text{Therefore } \% \text{ solution} \times \text{volume} = \frac{\text{weight} \times 100}{\text{volume}} \times \text{volume}$$

Volume can be cancelled out from the right hand side of the equation.

$$\text{Therefore } \% \text{ solution} \times \text{ volume} = \text{weight} \times 100$$

The next step is to remove the 100 from the right hand side of the equation by dividing both sides by 100.

$$\text{Therefore } \frac{\% \text{ solution} \times \text{volume}}{100} = \frac{\text{weight} \times 100}{100}$$

Now 100 can be removed from the right hand side by cancelling out.

$$\text{Therefore } \frac{\% \text{ solution} \times \text{volume}}{100} = \text{weight}$$

$$\text{e.g. weight of solution y} = \frac{5 \times 750}{100} = \textbf{37.5 g}$$

Table **2.2** Examples of percentage solutions

Solution	% solution	volume ml	weight g
y	5	750	37.5
x	2	1200	24
z	4	800	32

Example 4

A veterinary surgeon has analysed 'patients' over the last year and has created the following table from the data:

Table **2.3** Patients treated over the previous year

	Dogs	**Cats**	**Birds**	**Exotics**	**TOTAL**
Jan–Mar	260	150	90	28	528
Apr–Jun	329	192	71	19	611
Jul–Sep	197	201	52	21	471
Oct–Dec	419	157	87	32	695
Totals	1205	700	300	100	**2305**

(i) What is the percentage of each category of birds and animals treated?
(ii) In which quarter does the percentage of exotics treated exceed 5% of the total animals treated in that quarter?
(iii) Convert the above table into percentages using the total 2305 as the base.

Calculations:

(i) Calculations to find the % of each category of animal

$$\text{Dogs} \quad \frac{1205 \times 100}{2305} = 52.28\%$$

$$\text{Cats} \quad \frac{700 \times 100}{2305} = 30.37\%$$

$$\text{Birds} \quad \frac{300 \times 100}{2305} = 13.02\%$$

$$\text{Exotics} \quad \frac{100 \times 100}{2305} = 4.34\%$$

(ii)   To calculate the percentage of exotics treated each quarter, compile a simple table as set out below :

Quarter	Number of exotics treated	Total animals treated per quarter	% of exotics treated in quarter
1	28	528	5.30
2	19	611	3.11
3	21	471	4.46
4	32	695	4.60

From the table it can be seen that the number of exotics treated exceeds 5% of the total animals treated during the first quarter of the year.

(iii)   Calculations to find the % of each category of animal treated per quarter. Example of a calculation given in table 2.4:

$$\text{Dogs 1st quarter:} \quad \frac{260}{2305} \times 100 = 11.28\%$$

Table 2.4 Percentage of animals treated per quarter

	Dogs	**Cats**	**Birds**	**Exotics**	**TOTAL**
Jan–Mar	11.28	6.51	3.90	1.21	22.91
Apr–Jun	14.27	8.33	3.08	0.82	26.51
Jul–Sep	8.55	8.72	2.26	0.91	20.43
Oct–Dec	18.18	6.81	3.77	1.39	30.15
Totals	52.28	30.37	13.02	4.34	**100.00**

Self-test exercise 6
(answers at the end of this chapter)

Calculate the percentages for each of the cell types from the three batches of differential white blood cell counts, which are listed in the following table, and then complete the table. Round the percentages to the nearest whole number.

Table 2.5 Differential leucocyte counts

Batch No.	Type 1	Type 2	Type 3	Type 4	Type 5	Total cell count
No. 2	29	14	11	14	6	74
Type %						
No. 3	26	14	10	27	9	86
Type %						
No. 4	22	10	7	13	3	55
Type %						

(ii)   The dose of a drug, which is currently given at 200 mg per day is to be reduced by 20%. What will the new daily dose be?
(iii) What percentage of 500 mg is 50 mg?
(iv)   A drug has to be given five times per day. What percentage of the daily total is each dose?

Manipulation of formulae (equations)

There are many occasions when a simple equation has to be changed around (or transposed) so that it can be applied to a practical problem. For example, if $A = B \times C$ and the value of B has to be calculated, the equation has to be transposed so that it makes B the *subject* of the equation.

In this case, $B = \dfrac{A}{C}$ (This is explained later in this chapter)

As a practical example of the above, suppose that a certain drug had to be administered at a rate of 20 mg per kg of body weight. If the body weight were 12 kg, the total dose would be 240 mg.

Expressing the above information as a simple equation (or formula) it can be stated that:

Total dose = dose rate × body weight
i.e. 240 mg = 20 mg/kg × 12 kg

If the situation were changed so that it were necessary to calculate what weight of animal the same total amount of drug would be suitable for, then the equation would have to be transposed in order to make body weight the subject.

In this case body weight $= \dfrac{\text{total dose}}{\text{dose rate}}$

(see below for explanation, rules 1 and 3)

Basic mathematical rules

There are some basic rules that must be adhered to when using or transposing equations of any kind. An equation is exactly what it says it is, i.e. *equal*. It is imperative that it remains equal no matter what is done to it.

Rule 1

Whatever happens to the left hand side must also happen to the right hand side.

Therefore, taking the equation $A + B = C$ as an example, if the left hand side is multiplied by 2, to keep the equation *equal*, the right hand side must also be multiplied by 2.

The equation becomes $2 \times (A + B) = 2 \times C$

Notice also that if the figures on one side of the equation are added together like A and B in the example, then they *must* have a bracket put round them before they can be multiplied by the 2.

The same principle applies if the left hand side is divided by 2. In this case, the right hand side of the equation must also be divided by 2 in order to keep the equation *equal* (or balanced).

So, the equation would become $\dfrac{(A + B)}{2} = \dfrac{C}{2}$

To prove the above, replace A, B and C by easy numbers that can be worked out mentally. For instance, if A is 2 and B is 4 then C must be 6. Putting these into the original equation would give $2 + 4 = 6$ which is clearly the right answer. If the right hand side is multiplied by 2 then the left hand side must also be multiplied by 2 to keep the equation in balance.

$2 \times (2 + 4) = 2 \times 6$ would give $12 = 12$

However, if the brackets had been omitted on the left hand side it would be easy to miscalculate as follows:

$2 \times 2 + 4 = 2 \times 6$

This would give $4 + 4 = 12$ which is clearly a nonsense.

Division works in exactly the same way. If one side of the equation is divided by 2 then the other side must *also* be divided by 2.

Replacing A, B and C with the same simple numbers proves the point. If $A = 2$, $B = 4$ and $C = 6$,

$$\frac{(2 + 4)}{2} = \frac{6}{2}$$

Therefore $\dfrac{6}{2} = \dfrac{6}{2}$

Therefore $3 = 3$

Rule 2

To change sides, change signs.

Using the same simple example of $A + B = C$, in order to change the equation to make A the *subject* i.e. so that it reads $A =$, as opposed to $A + B =$, then the B on the left hand side must be 'disposed of'. The only place it can go is to the other side of the equation. Taking the B to the other side involves changing its sign from $+B$ to $-B$. Therefore $A = C - B$.

Again, this can be proven by replacing the letters with the same numbers that were used in the previous examples.

Therefore $2 = 6 - 4$

Rule 3

Fractional equations can be cross-multiplied.

Fractional equations such as $\dfrac{A}{B} = \dfrac{C}{D}$ can be simplified using a technique known as cross-multiplication. This involves multiplying the bottom of the left hand side by the top of the right hand side and multiplying the bottom of the right hand side by the top of the left hand side. In the above example, after cross-multiplication the equation becomes:

$A \times D = B \times C$

In order to make A the subject and dispose of D on the left hand side, divide both sides by D:

Therefore $\dfrac{A \times D}{D} = \dfrac{B \times C}{D}$

The Ds on the left hand side can also be cancelled:

Therefore $\dfrac{A \times 1}{1} = \dfrac{B \times C}{D}$ but, $\dfrac{A \times 1}{1} = A$

Therefore $A = \dfrac{B \times C}{D}$

To make B, C, or D the subject, exactly the same process is followed.

Answers to self-test exercises

Exercise 1

(i) 5   (ii) $\frac{1}{2}$ (iii) 3   (iv) $\frac{3}{4}$ (v) $\frac{1}{3}$
(vi) $4\frac{1}{2}$ (vii) $\frac{1}{2}$ (viii) $1\frac{1}{3}$ (ix) 3   (x) 28

Exercise 2

(i) 0.5   (ii) 0.5   (iii) 0.63   (iv) 0.33   (v) 1.82
(vi) 0.75   (vii) 0.6   (viii) 0.44   (ix) 0.79   (x) 0.32

Exercise 3

(i) 10   (ii) 9   (iii) 9
(iv) 9.9   (v) 9.1   (vi) 9.0
(vii) 9.88   (viii) 9.09   (ix) 9.01

Exercise 4

(i) 500, 50, 5, 0.5
(ii) 5000, 500, 50, 5
(iii) 50 000, 5000, 500, 50
(iv) 600, 0.6, 0.06, 0.006
(v) 60, 0.06, 0.006, 0.0006
(vi) 6, 0.006, 0.0006, 0.00006

Exercise 5

(i) 50%   (ii) 50%   (iii) 158.33%   (iv) 75%
(v) 182.35%   (vi) 75%   (vii) 23.08%
(viii) 33.33%   (ix) 46.15%   (x) 38.23%

Exercise 6

(i)   see table below

Table 2.6 Differential leucocyte counts

Batch No.	Type 1	Type 2	Type 3	Type 4	Type 5	Total cell count
No. 2	29	14	11	14	6	74
Type %	39	19	15	19	8	
No. 3	26	14	10	27	9	86
Type %	30	16	12	31	10	
No. 4	22	10	7	13	3	55
Type %	40	18	13	24	5	

(ii)   160 mg
(iii)   10%
(iv)   20%

Chapter 3

Changing the Concentration of a Solution

This is a very practical problem, as concentrated solutions are often the preferred method of transportation, leaving the veterinary practice to dilute them to the strength required. Conversely, there may be instances where the only solution available is weaker than the one required and the solution has to be more concentrated. There are several methods of approaching the problem of changing the concentration of solutions. Therefore, where appropriate, at least one alternative method of performing the calculations has been illustrated in this chapter.

Notes

- The standard formula for a percentage solution

$$= \frac{\textbf{weight of substance in grams (solute)}}{\textbf{volume of water in millilitres (solvent)}} \times \textbf{100}$$

- The above formula is often written as:

  % solution = weight (in g)/volume (in ml) × 100

- When % solution is written in the above form, *the forward slash indicates 'over' or a fraction*

Example 1

(i)   20 g dissolved in 100 ml
      $= 20/100 \times 100\% = \mathbf{20\%}$

(ii) 25 g dissolved in 400 ml
      $= 25/400 \times 100\% = \mathbf{6.25\%}$

(iii) 30 g dissolved in 1000 ml
      $= 30/1000 \times 100 = \mathbf{3\%}$

Dilution of a concentrated solution

Example 2

A 50% solution of a particular drug is available at the practice. 500 ml of a 2.5% solution of this drug is required. Calculate the amount of the 50% solution and additional water that is required.

Summary of facts relating to this problem

$$\textbf{\% solution} = \frac{\textbf{weight in g}}{\textbf{volume in ml}} \times \textbf{100}$$

(or weight in g/volume in ml $\times 100$)

Therefore a 50% solution $= 50\,\text{g}/100\,\text{ml} \times 100$

$$= \frac{50\,\text{g}}{100\,\text{ml}} \times 100$$

Likewise a 2.5% solution $= 2.5\,\text{g}/100\,\text{ml} \times 100$

$$= \frac{2.5\,\text{g}}{100\,\text{ml}} \times 100$$

Answer

Method 1

To use the more concentrated 50% solution to make a 2.5% solution, find out how many ml of the 50% solution contains

2.5 g of the drug (solute). Once this is known it is easier to change the 50% solution into the required solution strength.

Why 2.5 g? Because that is the weight of the solute required in every 100 ml of a 2.5% solution.

100 ml of a 50% solution contains 50 g of drug.

But only 2.5 g of drug are required in the 2.5% solution.

That is only $\frac{2.5}{50}$ or $\frac{1}{20}$ of the amount.

$\frac{1}{20}$ of the drug will be contained in $\frac{1}{20}$ of the volume of the 50% solution.

Therefore, the volume of the 50% solution which contains 2.5 g of drug will be $\frac{100}{20} = 5$ ml.

Therefore, to produce a 2.5% solution (which is 2.5 g in 100 ml of solution), for each 100 ml of a 2.5% solution required take:

5 ml of the 50% solution plus 95 ml of sterile water
= 100 ml of 2.5% solution

Originally, the question asked for 5 times this amount, i.e. 500 ml of a 2.5% solution of this drug. Therefore:

5 ml of the 50% solution is multiplied by 5 = 25 ml
Plus,
95 ml of the sterile water is multiplied by 5 = 475 ml
= **500 ml of a 2.5% solution**

Method 2

Rather than performing the calculation from first principles as shown in method 1, the volume of the solution available which must be used to obtain a specified dilution can be found by applying the following formula:

$$\frac{\textbf{strength required}}{\textbf{strength available}} \times \textbf{final volume}$$

Therefore volume of the 50% solution required

$$= \frac{2.5}{50} \times 500 \, \text{ml} = 25 \, \text{ml}$$

Therefore, to make 500 ml of 2.5 % solution, *take 25 ml of the 50% solution and make it up to 500 ml with 475 ml of sterile water.*

Example 3

Once again a 50% solution is available. This time, 500 ml of a 10% solution is required from it. What needs to be done to complete this task?

Answer

Method 1

A 50% solution is available. This can be expressed as $50\,g/100\,ml \times 100$. 500 ml of a 10% solution is required. In standard form, a 10% solution can be expressed as $10\,g/100\,ml \times 100$. This time, the volume of the 50% solution which contains 10 g of drug has to be calculated first.

50 g are contained in 100 ml.
Therefore, 10 g (which is $\frac{1}{5}$ of 50) will be contained in $\frac{1}{5}$ of $100\,ml = 20\,ml$

Therefore, 20 ml of the 50% solution made up to 100 ml with sterile water will produce 100 ml of 10% solution.

The question requires that 500 ml of the solution be produced, and 20 ml of the 50% solution is required to make 100 ml of 10% solution. *Therefore 100 ml of the 50% solution will have to be made up to 500 ml with 400 ml of sterile water in order to make 500 ml of 10% solution i.e. $100 \times 5 = 500\,ml$.*

Method 2

$$\frac{\textbf{strength required}}{\textbf{strength available}} \times \textbf{final volume}$$

Therefore volume of the 50% solution required

$$= \frac{10}{50} \times 500\,\text{ml} = 100\,\text{ml}$$

Therefore, 100 ml of the 50% solution will have to be made up to 500 ml with 400 ml of sterile water in order to make 500 ml of 10% solution.

Example 4

This example is a more complex variation of examples 2 and 3 (the answer is based on method 1 shown in examples 2 and 3). 500 ml of a 20% solution is available in the drug store.

(i)   Two solutions are required as follows:

> Solution 1 requires 200 ml of a 2.5% solution
> Solution 2 requires 500 ml of a 1% solution

What calculations are needed to produce the two required solutions from the 20% solution?

(ii)   What volume would remain of the original 20% solution?

(iii) What weight of solute would be in the remaining volume?

Answer

(i)   *What calculations are needed to produce the two required solutions from the 20% solution?*

Given solution: 500 ml of 20% solution is available.
A standard 20% solution is expressed as 20 g of solute in 100 ml of solvent (the base solution e.g. sterile water).
Therefore, there are 5×20 g in 5×100 ml of this solution, i.e. 100 g in 500 ml.
Solution 1 requires 200 ml of a 2.5% solution.
A standard 2.5% solution is expressed as 2.5 g of solute in 100 ml of solvent.

Therefore, there are 2×2.5 g in 2×100 ml of this solution, i.e. 5 g in 200 ml.

Solution 2 requires 500 ml of a 1% solution.

A standard 1% solution is expressed as 1 g in 100 ml of solvent. Therefore, there are 5×1 g in 5×100 ml of this solution, i.e. 5 g in 500 ml.

Calculate how many ml of the more concentrated 20% solution contains 5 g of the solute.

It is known that there are 100 g of solute in 500 ml = 20%

Only 5 g are required to make 500 ml of a 1% solution, therefore $\dfrac{100\,\text{g}}{5\,\text{g}} = 20$ i.e. 5 g is $\frac{1}{20}$ of 100 g

Then the 5 g will be contained in $\dfrac{500\,\text{ml}}{20\,\text{ml of solution}} = 25\,\text{ml}$

i.e. **5 g are contained in 25 ml of solution**

Solution 1

Take 25 ml of the 20% solution and add 175 ml of solvent (e.g. sterile water)

$= 5$ g in (25 ml + 175 ml = 200 ml)

i.e. 5 g in 200 ml $= \dfrac{5\,\text{g}}{200\,\text{ml}} \times 100\%$

$\qquad\qquad = \textbf{2.5\% solution}$

Solution 2

Take 25 ml of the 20% solution and add 475 ml of solvent (e.g. sterile water)

$= 5$ g in (25 ml + 475 ml = 500 ml)

i.e. 5 g in 500 ml $= \dfrac{5\,\text{g}}{500\,\text{ml}} \times 100\%$

$\qquad\qquad = \textbf{1\% solution}$

(ii)   *What volume would remain of the original 20% solution?*

Answer $= 500\,\text{ml} - 2 \times 25\,\text{ml samples}$

$\qquad\quad = \textbf{450 ml}$

(iii) *What weight of solute would be in the remaining volume?*

Weight of solute left in this 450 ml of 20% solution?

Original solution contained 100 g and 2 samples have been taken out containing 5 g.

Therefore, there must be 100 g − (2 samples × 5 g) = 90 g left.

Alternatively the answer could be calculated thus:

$$\% \text{ solution} = \frac{\text{weight}}{\text{volume}} \times 100 \text{ becomes:}$$

$$\text{weight} = \frac{\% \text{ solution} \times \text{volume}}{100}$$

$$\text{weight} = \frac{20 \times 450}{100} = \textbf{90 g}$$

Manipulating the formula (see also Chapter 2, Basic Principles)

The standard equation for a percentage solution is:

$$\% \text{ solution} = \text{weight in g/volume in ml} \times 100$$

$$\textbf{i.e. \% solution} = \frac{\textbf{weight in g}}{\textbf{volume in ml}} \times \textbf{100}$$

It is possible to manipulate this standard % solution formula to find the 'missing part'.

For example

$$\% \text{ solution} = \frac{\text{weight in g}}{\text{volume in ml}} \times 100 \qquad \text{(standard formula)}$$

$$\text{volume in ml} = \frac{\text{weight in g} \times 100}{\% \text{ solution}} \qquad \text{(manipulated formula)}$$

$$\text{weight in g} = \frac{\text{volume in ml} \times \% \text{ solution}}{100}$$

(manipulated formula)

It may be easier to remember the above manipulation if it is thought of as a triangle:

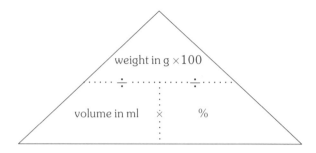

To apply the triangle:

- First put the known information into the appropriate places in the triangle
- Next, cover the part of the triangle which contains the information which has to be found
- Finally, divide or multiply (as appropriate) the remaining visible figures.

Example 5

Calculate the weight of solute which must be dissolved in 250 ml of solvent in order to make a 5% solution.

Answer

Place the known information in the appropriate parts of the triangle and cover the section marked 'weight' as shown below:

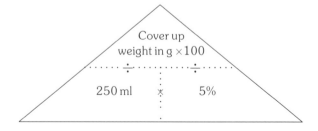

From the triangle, weight $\times$ 100 $=$ vol $\times$ %

$$\text{Therefore weight} \times 100 = 250 \times 5$$
$$= \mathbf{1250\,g}$$

In order to make weight the subject of the equation, i.e. to remove the 100 from the left hand side, both sides must be divided by 100.

$$\text{Therefore } \frac{\text{weight} \times 100}{100} = \frac{1250}{100} \text{ g}$$
$$\text{Therefore weight} = \mathbf{12.5\,g}$$

Example 6

Calculate what volume of a 25% solution contains 20 g of solute.

Answer

Place the known information in the appropriate parts of the triangle and cover section marked volume as shown below:

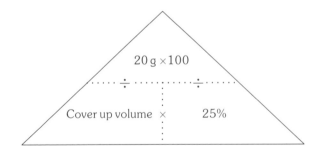

From the triangle, volume $= \dfrac{\text{weight} \times 100}{\%}$

$$= \frac{20 \times 100}{25} \text{ ml}$$
$$= \mathbf{80\,ml}$$

Example 7

What is the concentration of a solution which is produced by dissolving 15 g of solute in 60 ml of solvent?

Answer

Place the known information in the appropriate parts of the triangle and cover section marked % as shown below:

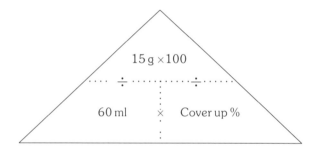

From the triangle % solution $= \dfrac{\text{weight} \times 100}{\text{volume}}$

$$= \dfrac{1500}{60}\%$$

$$= \mathbf{25\%}$$

Example 8

10 litres of a 25% solution are held in stock.
Earlier in the book, 250 ml of a 5% solution had been prepared from the above solution.

(i)   What weight of solute did this volume contain?
(ii) What volume of the 25% solution was used?
(iii) What amount of sterile water was added to reduce the concentration to 5%?

This question can easily be answered by using the standard formula for % solutions and by *manipulating the formula*:
Standard formula:

$$\% \text{ solution} = \frac{\text{weight in g}}{\text{volume in ml}} \times 100$$

For the 5% solution manipulate the formula to give:

$$\text{weight in g} = \frac{\% \text{ solution} \times \text{volume in ml}}{100}$$

Substituting the figures given means that the weight will be calculated first:

$$\text{weight in g} = \frac{5\% \times 250\,\text{ml}}{100} = 12.5\,\text{g}$$

i.e. weight of the solute in 250 ml = **12.5 g**

Now find what volume of the 25% solution contains 12.5 g of solute by substituting the values calculated

$$\text{volume} = \frac{12.5\,\text{g} \times 100}{25\%}$$
$$= \textbf{50\,ml}$$

250 ml of 5% solution was originally prepared from the stock solution. Therefore, **200 ml** needs to be added to this 50 ml.

Answers

(i)	Volume of the 25% solution used	= **50 ml**
(ii)	Weight this volume contains	= **12.5 g**
(iii)	Volume of sterile water added to give a 5% solution	= **200 ml**

Example 9

A surgery has run out of 5% solution of a drug. The veterinary surgeon has, however, requested that 250 ml of this solution be available for urgent treatment of a cat. There is only 500 ml of a

1.5% solution. Explain how 250 ml of 5% solution could be produced from the 1.5% stock.

Answer

To increase the concentration of a solution the weight of solute in a given volume of solvent must be increased.

The first step is to calculate the weight of the solute in 250 ml of the available solution.

Why 250 ml? This is the volume requested by the veterinary surgeon. Using the standard formula

$$\% \text{ solution} = \frac{\text{weight} \times 100}{\text{volume}}$$

and by manipulating it to give the *weight* as the *subject* of the equation:

$$\text{weight in g} = \frac{\% \text{ solution} \times \text{volume in ml}}{100}$$

By halving the volume of the available 1.5% solution to 250 ml, two parts of the equation are known.

The third unknown part can be calculated thus.

Substituting the 1.5% and the 250 ml into the equation gives the following:

$$\text{weight} = \frac{1.5\% \times 250 \text{ ml}}{100}$$
$$= 3.75 \text{ g in 250 ml of the 1.5\% solution}$$

If the same equation is used, but this time substituting the vet's requirements, the calculation becomes:

$$\text{weight} = \frac{5\% \times 250 \text{ ml}}{100}$$
$$= 12.5 \text{ g}$$

The situation can be recorded as follows:

Required weight of solute in 250 ml of 5% solution is 12.5 g
Actual weight of solute in 250 ml of 1.5% solution is 3.75 g

By adding (12.5 g – 3.75 g) = 8.75 g to 250 ml of the available 1.5% solution, the concentration can be increased from 1.5% to 5%. The standard formula can prove this: by substituting the known weight and volume values, the concentration can be calculated.

$$\text{Hence \% solution} = \frac{12.5\,\text{g} \times 100}{250\,\text{ml}} = 5\%$$

Self-test exercise
(fully-worked answers at the end of this chapter)

Changing the percentage concentration of a solution

(i)   (a)   How many grams of glucose powder are required to make 50 ml of a 2.5% solution?

       (b)   What weight of glucose should be added to increase the concentration of 50 ml of 2.5% solution (in (a)) to 5%?

(ii)   How much of 50% dextrose solution must be added to a 750 ml bag of sterile water (once an identical volume of water is removed) to make a 5% dextrose solution?

(iii) How many milligrams of solute are required to make 50 ml of 2.5% solution and what volume of sterile water is needed to reduce its concentration to a 0.25% solution?

(iv) Two solutions containing the same drug are mixed together. What is the resultant concentration if the two solutions are:
200 ml of 2% solution and 100 ml of 1% solution?

(v)   By adding 5 g of a solute to 200 ml of 3% solution containing the same solute, what is the % concentration of the new solution?

(vi) How much sterile liquid needs to be added to 100 ml of 10% solution to reduce its concentration by half?

(vii)   12 mg of a drug are dissolved in 50 ml of sterile fluid and 25 ml then used for an injection.
A further 25 ml of sterile fluid are then added to the unused 25 ml of original solution.
Calculate the % concentration of the final solution.

(viii)   When 250 ml of a 20% solution were accidentally added to a 750 ml beaker of sterile water the vet, who had asked for 250 ml of a 5% solution, was not concerned. Why?

(ix)   10 mg of a drug are dissolved in 5 ml of a sterile fluid but the required concentration should have been 2.5%. What needs to be done to rectify the situation?

(x)   Four students have just finished working with the same solution in different concentrations. The laboratory technician has only one 5 litre beaker in which to keep all of the solutions left by the students. The technician decides to make up 2.5 litres of a 2.5% solution, in order to make stock-keeping simple. What must the technician do in order to accomplish this? Given that:

> Student 1 left 250 ml of a 5.0% solution
> Student 2 left 100 ml of a 10.0% solution
> Student 3 left 750 ml of a 2.5% solution
> Student 4 left 50 ml of a 1.0% solution

Answers to self-test exercises

(i)   Weight of glucose powder in 50 ml of 2.5% solution:
Use either the triangle diagram or the manipulated formula

$$\text{weight in g} = \frac{\text{volume in ml} \times \% \text{ solution}}{100}$$

Substituting known values gives:

$$\text{weight in g} = \frac{2.5\% \times 50\,\text{ml}}{100} = \mathbf{1.25\,g}$$

Use the same formula to calculate the weight of glucose in 50 ml of a 5% solution.

$$\text{weight in g} = \frac{5.0\% \times 50\,\text{ml}}{100} = \textbf{2.5\,g}$$

Therefore to convert 50 ml of a 2.5% solution into 50 ml of a 5% solution, a further 1.25 g of glucose needs to be added to the 2.5% solution.

(ii) This question starts with 750 ml of sterile water in a bag. It then asks how much water needs to be removed and replaced by a dextrose solution to produce 750 ml of 5% solution of dextrose and then states that the only source of dextrose available is in a 50% solution. The first stage in calculating the answer to this question is to calculate the weight of dextrose needed to create 750 ml of 5% solution.

$$\text{Use weight in g} = \frac{750\,\text{ml} \times 5\%}{100} = 37.5\,\text{g of dextrose}$$

The only source of dextrose available is a 50% concentrated solution. Therefore what volume of 50% solution contains 37.5 g of dextrose?

$$50\% \text{ solution} = \frac{50\,\text{g}}{100\,\text{ml}} \times 100$$

means that 1 g is dissolved in every 2 ml.

Therefore, what volume in ml of 50% solution contains 37.5 g of dextrose? If 1 g of a 50% solution is dissolved in 2 ml (see above), then 37.5 g of dextrose will be dissolved, or contained in, 37.5×2 ml $= 75$ ml. Therefore, if 75 ml of sterile water are taken out of the bag containing 750 ml, leaving 675 ml of sterile water, and 75 ml of a 50% solution of dextrose are added to the 675 ml of sterile water, then the resulting solution will contain 37.5 g of dextrose.

This means that the resulting solution will have 37.5 g of solute in 750 ml of solution.

Using the equation

$$\% \text{ solution} = \frac{\text{weight in g}}{\text{volume in ml}} \times 100$$

to check the concentration of the new mixture gives the following answer:

$$\% \text{ solution} = \frac{37.5\,\text{g}}{750\,\text{ml}} \times 100 = 5\%$$

(iii) This question is best answered by first calculating the weight of solute in the 2.5% solution using the standard formula and substituting the known values:

$$\text{weight in g} = \frac{2.5\% \times 50\,\text{ml}}{100} = 1.25\,\text{g}$$

Expressed in mg this is $(1.25 \times 1000)\,\text{mg} = 1250\,\text{mg}$

The question then asks how this solution can be diluted to change it into a 0.25% strength solution.

This requires the weight to volume ratio of the above solution to be calculated.

In other words, how many g of solute are contained in a standard 0.25% solution, again using the standard formula:

$$\% \text{ solution} = \frac{\text{weight in g}}{\text{volume in ml}} \times 100$$

$$0.25\% \text{ solution} = \frac{0.25\,\text{g}}{100\,\text{ml}} \times 100 = 0.25\,\text{g in } 100 \text{ ml}$$

or it can also be expressed as $(0.25 \times 1000)\,\text{mg}$ in 100 ml

or as the ratio of 250 mg of solute in 100 ml of solution producing a solution of 0.25% concentration.

Two sets of data have now been calculated from the data given in the question.

50 ml of a 2.5% solution contain 1250 mg of solute.

(*statement 1*)

100 ml of a 0.25% solution contain 250 mg of the same solute (*statement 2*)

The question asks, 'What volume of sterile water is needed to reduce the concentration of the 2.5% solution to a 0.25% solution?'

In order to compare the two solutions, either the weights or the volumes need to be equal.

In this case, as the question requires the 2.5% solution to be diluted i.e. volume added by the addition of more water, the weight needs to remain constant.

To do this, statement 2 needs to be multiplied by 5 to get the weight the same as in statement 1.

i.e. 5×100 ml of a 0.25% solution contain 5×250 mg of solute which translates to 500 ml of a 0.25% solution contain 1250 mg of solute.

Comparing this to statement 1 which is:

50 ml of a 2.5% solution contain 1250 mg of solute

The question asks 'what volume of sterile water is needed?' By deduction, if 50 ml of a 2.5% solution contain 1250 mg of solute and 500 ml of 0.25% solution contain 1250 mg of the same solute, then the addition of $(500 - 50 =)450$ ml of sterile water to the 2.5% solution will give a 0.25% solution.

(iv) The key to answering this question is to calculate the weight of the solute in each of the given solutions. Add the weights together and divide the weight by the total volume using the standard formula for a % solution to calculate the new concentration.

Use the manipulated formula

$$\text{weight in g} = \frac{2\% \times 200\,\text{ml}}{100} = 4\,\text{g}$$

and for the other solution,

$$\text{weight in g} = \frac{1\% \times 100\,\text{ml}}{100} = 1\,\text{g}$$

Add the two weights to give 5 g, and the two volumes $(200 + 100) = 300\,\text{ml}$.

Use the standard formula

$$\% \text{ solution} = \frac{\text{weight in g}}{\text{volume in ml}} \times 100$$

Substitute known values

$$\% \text{ solution} = \frac{5\,\text{g}}{300\,\text{ml}} \times 100 = \textbf{1.67\% solution}$$

(v)   To answer this question, use the manipulated formula to calculate the weight of solute in the given solution. Then add 5 g to the weight calculated. Recalculate using the standard formula with the new values.

Use manipulated formula

$$\text{weight in g} = \frac{\% \text{ solution} \times \text{volume in ml}}{100}$$

Substitute given values

$$\text{Weight in g} = \frac{3\% \times 200\,\text{ml}}{100} = 6\,\text{g}$$

Add 5 g to give 11 g
Recalculate using standard formula

$$\% \text{ solution} = 11\,\text{g in } 200\,\text{ml} \times 100 = \textbf{5.5\%}$$

Note: only the weight changes, not the volume.

(vi) The technique for answering this question is exactly the same as those above. Use the standard formula to express each of the solutions by weight and volume. Thus a 10% standard solution is:

$$10\% \text{ solution} = \frac{10\,\text{g}}{100\,\text{ml}} \times 100$$

$$5\% \text{ solution} = \frac{5\,\text{g}}{100\,\text{ml}} \times 100$$

or, it can also be expressed as $\dfrac{10\,\text{g}}{200\,\text{ml}}$ by multiplying top and bottom of the equation by 2.

This enables direct comparison of the 10% and the 5% solutions as both have the same weight but are dissolved in different volumes. Hence:

10% solution is 10 g of solute dissolved in 100 ml of solution
5% solution is 10 g of solute dissolved in 200 ml of solution

Adding **100 ml** of sterile liquid to a 10% solution would convert it to a 5% solution.

(vii) This question is similar to question (v) except that the volume changes rather than the weight.

12 mg of drug are dissolved in 50 ml of sterile fluid.

25 ml are used for an injection.

This leaves 25 ml of the solution (i.e. half) containing 6 mg of solute, i.e. half of the weight.

A further 25 ml of fluid are added.

Which gives 6 mg in (25 ml + 25 ml =) 50 ml of solution.

Use the standard formula to calculate the concentration after changing the weight units to g (as the standard requires).

$$6\,\text{mg} = \frac{6}{1000\,\text{g}} = 0.006\,\text{g}$$

$$\%\text{ solution} = \frac{0.006\,\text{g}}{50\,\text{ml}} \times 100 = \textbf{0.012\% solution}$$

(viii) This question can only be answered by using the standard calculation for a % solution to determine the weight in the 20% solution, then adding 750 ml of volume to the solution, and recalculating using the standard formula.

Using manipulated formula

$$\text{weight in g} = \frac{\% \text{ solution} \times \text{volume in ml}}{100}$$

$$\text{weight in g} = \frac{20\% \times 250 \, \text{ml}}{100} = 50 \, \text{g}$$

The weight is now known. The volume was 250 ml and has been increased by being accidentally added to a beaker containing 750 ml of sterile water, i.e. the total volume has increased to (250 ml + 750 ml =) 1000 ml of solution.

The concentration is now $= \dfrac{50 \, \text{g}}{1000 \, \text{ml}} \times 100 = 5\%$

Exactly what the vet asked for, hence the lack of concern!

(ix)   First calculate the % concentration of the solution.
Note that the weight is in mg, and must be converted to g.
Then express 2.5% solution in standard terms.
Make either the weight or the volume equal in both solutions.
Compare the answers and deduce what has to be done to convert one solution into the other.
Calculate the % solution from the facts given in the question.

$$\% \text{ solution} = \frac{0.010 \, \text{g}}{5 \, \text{ml}} \times 100$$

(weight needs to be converted to g first)

$$= 0.2\%$$

$$2.5\% = \frac{2.5 \, \text{g}}{100 \, \text{ml}} \times 100$$

$$\text{or } 2.5\% = \frac{(2.5 \times 1000) \, \text{mg}}{100 \, \text{ml}} \times 100$$

$$\text{i.e. } 2.5\% = \frac{2500 \, \text{mg}}{100 \, \text{ml}} \times 100 \qquad (\textit{equation 1})$$

expressed as weight in mg in 5 ml (which is the volume of the original solution) gives $\dfrac{125 \, \text{mg}}{5 \, \text{ml}}$ (divide top and bottom of equation 1 by 20).

Therefore if 10 mg in 5 ml = 0.2% solution
and 125 mg in 5 ml = 2.5% solution
then **115 mg** (125 mg − 10 mg) **of solute must be added** to rectify the situation.

This will convert the 0.2% solution into a 2.5% solution

(x) In each case, the weight of solute in the solution left by the students must be calculated. Use the manipulated formula:

$$\text{weight in g} = \frac{\% \text{ solution} \times \text{volume in ml}}{100}$$

$$\text{Student 1 weight in solution} = \frac{5\% \times 250 \text{ ml}}{100} = 12.50 \text{ g}$$

$$\text{Student 2 weight in solution} = \frac{10\% \times 100 \text{ ml}}{100}$$

$$= 10.00 \text{ g}$$

$$\text{Student 3 weight in solution} = \frac{2.5\% \times 750 \text{ ml}}{100}$$

$$= 18.75 \text{ g}$$

$$\text{Student 4 weight in solution} = \frac{1.0\% \times 50 \text{ ml}}{100} = 0.50 \text{ g}$$

Total weight in solution is
41.75 g in (250 + 100 + 750 + 50 =)1150 ml

Using $\dfrac{\text{weight in g}}{\text{volume in ml}} \times 100$ and the figures above, the mixed solution has a combined concentration of $\dfrac{41.75 \text{ g}}{1150 \text{ ml}} \times 100 = 3.63\%$.

The technician wants to store this as 2.5 litres of a 2.5% solution.

The weight of solute in this solution can be calculated from the equation

$$\frac{2.5\% \times 2500 \text{ ml}}{100} = 62.5 \text{ g}$$

or 62.5 g dissolved in 2500 ml is equivalent to a 2.5% solution.

The mixture of the students' solutions gave $41.75\,g$ in $1150\,ml$.

Therefore the technician needs to add $(62.5\,g - 41.75\,g) = \mathbf{20.75\,g}$ to the solution and increase the volume to 2500 ml by adding $(2500\,ml - 1150\,ml) = \mathbf{1350\,ml}$ of sterile water.

To check this answer substitute the calculated figures into the standard formula.

$$\% \text{ solution} = \frac{41.75\,g + 20.75\,g}{1150\,ml + 1350\,ml} \times 100$$

$$= \frac{62.5\,g}{2500\,ml} \times 100 = 2.5\%$$

Chapter 4

Calculating Energy Requirements

In physics, 1 calorie is the amount of heat required to raise the temperature of 1 g of water by 1°C. More correctly, energy should be expressed in terms of joules. To convert calories to joules, multiply the calorie value by 4.2 (4.18 to be totally accurate).

However, energy in food is usually defined in both units, i.e. in kilojoules (kJ) and kilocalories (kcal). Calculations relating to food units usually use kilocalories, where one kilocalorie is equal to 1000 calories.

Thus 1 kilocalorie = 1000 calories.

Note

In this chapter there are several types of energy requirements but the unit used for all of them is the kcal.

Basal Energy Requirement – BER

This is the energy required by an animal (even when it is asleep) to sustain its Basal Metabolic Rate (BMR) generally calculated for a 24 hr period.

For dogs >5 kg (or >2 kg, in some publications)
The BER is calculated from the formula:
BER kcal = 30 × body weight + 70

For cats and small dogs
The BER is calculated using the formula:
BER kcal $= 60 \times$ body weight

Resting Energy Requirement – RER

This is the energy required by an animal at rest in an environment that is at the optimum temperature for the species.

The RER is calculated using the formula for BER.

Maintenance Energy Requirement – MER

This is the amount of energy used by an active animal in an optimum temperature for the species.

The MER is calculated from the formula:
MER kcal $=$ RER $\times 1.8$

Illness Energy Requirement – IER

This is the extra energy required by an animal in order to help it recover from trauma and/or repair damaged tissue.

To calculate the IER it is necessary to have access to a table of factors for various conditions. See table 4.1.

Table 4.1 Disease factors

Description	Disease factor
Cage rest	1.2
Surgery/trauma	1.3
Multiple surgery/trauma	1.5
Sepsis/neoplasia	1.7
Burns/scalding	2.0
Growth	2.0

Notes

- If the animal has multiple conditions, for example sepsis (1.7) and burns (2.0), the highest factor, in this example 2.0, is used.
- The factors are not added together or multiplied. The highest factor prevails. The IER is calculated from the formula:
  IER kcal = BER × disease factor
- Also note that the calculation results in the number of kcal required by the animal over a given time period.

Example 1

Calculate the RER for an adult cat with a body weight of 4 kg.

Answer

Using the formula:
RER kcal = 60 × body weight
And substituting the figure given for the cat's body weight (4 kg).
RER = 60 × 4 kcal = **240 kcal** in a 24 hour period

Example 2

Calculate the MER for a 60 kg Irish wolfhound.

Answer

In this example, the BER should be calculated first using the formula:

BER = 30 × body weight + 70 kcal for a 24 hour period.
Substituting the body weight of the hound into the formula gives
BER = 30 × 60 kg + 70 kcal for a 24 hour period
BER = 1800 + 70 = 1870 kcal for a 24 hour period

MER = 1.8 × BER
MER = 1.8 × 1870 kcal for a 24 hour period
MER = **3366 kcal** for a 24 hour period

Example 3

A 2.5 kg cat has been involved in a road traffic accident (RTA) and requires an operation to repair a fracture of both femurs. Calculate the IER.

Answer

Using the formula:
IER = BER × disease factor
BER = 60 × 2.5 kg = 150 kcal
IER = BER × disease factor
Substituting the calculated BER figure and the factor from the table above gives:
IER = 150 × 1.5 = **225 kcal**

Note

- From the table, the factors for both surgery and trauma (RTA) are 1.5, therefore the factor to use is 1.5, not 2 × 1.5 (= 3).

Self-test exercise

(i)   Calculate the RER for a 20 kg dog, a 5 kg cat and a 1 kg kitten.

(ii) Calculate the MER for the following:

   3 kg rabbit
   5 kg cat
   12 kg Basenji
   70 kg Irish wolfhound

(iii)   Calculate the IER for the patients listed below

A 20 kg dog has suffered multiple injuries in an RTA.
A 3 kg cat burnt in a house fire which develops infection in the wound within 1 week.
A 4 kg rabbit recovering from surgery needing cage rest.

Answers to self-test exercise

As these calculations are similar in nature they can be answered in tabular form.

Table 4.2 Answers to calculation of energy requirements

(i)

Patient	× Factor	Body weight kg	Additional factor	Total kcal
Dog	30	20	70	670
Cat	60	5	–	300
Kitten	60	1	–	60

Table 4.3 Answers to calculation of energy requirements

(ii)

Patient	× Factor	Body weight kg	Additional factor	Constant factor	Total kcal
Rabbit	60	3	–	1.8	324
Cat	60	5	–	1.8	540
Basenji	30	12	70	1.8	774
Irish wolfhound	30	70	70	1.8	3906

Table 4.4 Answers to calculation of energy requirements

(iii)

Patient	× Factor	Body weight kg	Additional factor	Disease factor	Total kcal
Dog	30	20	70	1.5	1005
Cat	60	3	–	2.0	360
Rabbit	60	4	–	1.3	312

Chapter 5

Dosages – Oral Route

These extremely important calculations relate a drug dosage to an animal's body weight and the period of time over which it is administered. Thus, the dose rate is normally expressed in the following units: mg/kg/day. That is, mg per kg of the drug to be given, multiplied by the animal's body weight in kg, to be administered over a given time period. There is always a time element involved, such as twice daily (b.i.d.) or 'x' number of tablets, say, every 8 hours (hrs).

The body weight may need to be converted from lb to kg. From the conversion tables within this book, it can be determined that: 2.2 lb converts to 1 kg. If such conversions are needed in an examination, multiples of 11 lb are often used to make the figures easier to convert.

It follows therefore that 22 lb is equal to 10 kg (just multiply each side of the equation by 10). Therefore, a 22 lb dog becomes a 10 kg dog and a 44 lb dog becomes a 20 kg dog. See table 5.1.

Table 5.1 Conversion of lb to kg

lb	kg
22	10
33	15
44	20
55	25
66	30

The dosages calculated can be either in solid form as a tablet, or in liquid form which is administered with a graduated dropper or syringe.

Example 1

A 5 kg rabbit requires medication at the rate of 50 mg/kg per day and the total amount should be split into two doses. A liquid form for oral dosage is available at 125 mg per ml.

How many ml should be administered to the rabbit over the course of the day?

Answer

Body weight of rabbit = 5 kg
Dose rate/kg of body weight = 50 mg
Dose = body weight in kg × dose rate in mg/kg of body weight

$$= 5 \text{ kg} \times 50 \text{ mg/kg}$$
$$= 250 \text{ mg}$$

NB: the kg cancel out and the answer is left in mg
1 ml contains 125 mg of antibiotic
Therefore, the number of ml required per day

$$= \frac{250 \text{ mg}}{125 \text{ mg}} = \textbf{2 ml}$$

Therefore the dose of 250 mg should be given as 1 ml b.i.d.

Example 2

A dog weighing 88 lb needs a course of antibiotics, which are available as 100 mg tablets.
The recommended daily dose is 10 mg/kg of body weight.

(a) How many tablets are required?
(b) What would the tablet requirement be if it was a puppy weighing 22 lb?

Answer

In this example, both answers can be calculated together

Body weight of dogs in lb	88	22
Body weight in kg	40	10
Dosage mg/kg	10	10
Dosage in mg	400	100
Tablet strength/mg	100	100
Tablets required	4	1

Notice however that the ratio of the dogs' weights is $88 : 22$ which is the same as $4 : 1$.

Once the tablet requirement had been calculated for the adult dog i.e. 4 tablets, the requirement for the puppy could be deduced i.e. 1 tablet.

As the dosage remains constant per kg of body weight, then the ratio of weights is reflected in the ratio of the tablets.

Example 3

A young Chihuahua weighs 2 kg and requires a drug at a dose rate of 4 mg/kg/day.

The tablet strength is 8 mg. How many tablets are required per dose if they are administered b.i.d.?

Answer

Body weight = 2 kg
Dose rate = 4 mg/kg
Dose calculated = 2 kg × 4 mg /kg = 8 mg
Tablet dose = 8 mg
Tablets required = $\dfrac{\text{calculated dose 8 mg}}{\text{tablet dose 8 mg}}$ = 1 tablet
Dosing period = b.i.d.
Dose/occasion = 1 tablet/2 occasions
            = $\frac{1}{2}$ **tablet b.i.d.**

Example 4

Antibiotics are to be given orally to a small goat weighing 4 kg. The dose rate is 50 mg/kg every 24 hours, for 7 days. The dose is to be divided so that it can be administered b.i.d.
How many ml of suspension should be dispensed if it contains 100 mg/ml of the antibiotic?

Answer

Body weight = 4 kg
Dose rate = 50 mg/kg
Dose calculated = 4 kg × 50 mg /kg = 200 mg/day
Suspension strength = 100 mg/ml
Volume required = $\dfrac{200\,\text{mg}}{100\,\text{mg}}$ = 2 ml/day
Dosing period = b.i.d.
ml/dose = 1 ml
Course of treatment for 7 days × 2 ml/day
Therefore, 14 ml should be dispensed.

Example 5

A dog weighs 35 kg and requires medication at a dose rate of 40 mg/kg.
The tablets available are 280 mg in strength.
How many tablets are required?
How would this dosage alter if the tablets were only 140 mg in strength?

Answer

Body weight = 35 kg
Dose rate = 40 mg/kg
Dose calculated = 35 kg × 40 mg/kg = 1400 mg
Tablet dose = 280 mg

Tablets required $= \dfrac{1400\,\text{mg}}{280\,\text{mg}} = 5$ tablets

If the tablets were only 140 mg in strength then the number of tablets would be $\dfrac{1400\,\text{mg}}{140\,\text{mg}} = \textbf{10 tablets}$.

Self-test exercise
(worked answers at the end of this chapter)

(i) A drug is available in tablets which should be administered at a dose rate of 3 mg/kg. This applies to all parts of the question.

 The tablets are to be given to an animal weighing 20 kg.
 (a) If the tablets available were 30 mg in strength, how many tablets does it need?
 (b) What would the requirement be if the tablet strength were 60 mg?

 The tablets are to be given to an animal weighing 60 kg.
 (c) If the tablets were 30 mg in strength, how many tablets would be required?
 (d) If the tablets were 20 mg in strength, how many tablets would be required?

(ii) A 20 kg animal requires a drug at the rate of 5 mg/kg/ 24 hrs. The drug is supplied as a 50 mg tablet. How many tablets are required for 7 days of treatment?

(iii) A 280 kg animal is receiving 4 tablets per day, for 7 days. The total daily dose is 560 mg. What is the:

 (a) weight of drug in each tablet?
 (b) dose rate in mg/kg/ 24 hrs?
 (c) total drug weight, in g, administered over the course of 7 days?

(iv) A hamster, weighing 125 g requires medication at the rate of 1 mg/kg of body weight per 8 hrs. An oral suspension is available containing 0.25 mg of drug per ml.

How many ml must be prescribed for a 7 day course of treatment?

(v) A 1 kg kitten requires 60 mg/kg/day of a drug.
The kitten has already had 8 tablets over the last 4 days.
The total course of treatment requires an intake of 0.3 g.
How many more days has the treatment to last before it is complete?
Each tablet contains 30 mg of drug.

(vi) A large bird weighing 33 lb is being treated with 2×12.5 mg tablets of a drug, b.i.d. The drug is administered in a food treat, over a 5 day period.
Calculate the daily dose rate in mg/kg.

What would the total dose of drug be for 5 days, if the bird weighed 44 lb and the dose rate remained the same?

(vii) How many tablets of 2.5 mg strength should be administered per dose to a 5 kg dog, if the dose rate is 4 mg/kg/day and the tablets are given b.i.d?

(viii) A 1500 g kitten needs 12 mg of a drug every 12 hours given in a 4 mg tablet form b.i.d.
Calculate the dose rate in mg/kg/day.

(ix) An animal is being treated with two 15 mg tablets every 8 hrs.
The dose rate is 5 mg/kg/day.
Which one of the following is the weight of the animal in kg?

(a) 12
(b) 16
(c) 18
(d) 20

(x) A 50 kg animal is being treated with 4 ml of antibiotic suspension every 6 hrs. Each ml of suspension contains 5 mg of drug.
Calculate the dose rate in mg/kg/day.

Answers to self-test exercise

(i) (a) Body weight of animal = 20 kg
Dose rate = 3 mg/kg
Dose required = 20 kg × 3 mg/kg = 60 mg
Each tablet contains 30 mg of the drug
Therefore number of tablets required = $\dfrac{60\,mg}{30\,mg}$
= **2 tablets**

(b) If the tablets were double the strength, i.e. 60 mg then only **1 tablet** would be required.

(c) However, if the animal to be treated weighed 60 kg and the dose rate remained the same at 3 mg/kg of body weight, the requirement would be 60 kg × 3 mg/kg = 180 mg.
If the tablets contained 30 mg of drug, then the number of tablets = $\dfrac{180\,mg}{30\,mg}$ = **6 tablets**

(d) For a drug requirement of 180 mg using 20 mg tablets, the number of tablets required = 180 mg/ 20 mg = **9 tablets**

(ii) Body weight of animal = 20 kg
Dose rate = 5 mg/kg/24 hrs
Requirement = 20 kg × 5 mg/kg = 100 mg
Each tablet contains 50 mg.
Therefore 2 tablets $\left(\dfrac{100\,mg}{50\,mg}\right)$ are required per day.
Consequently, **14 tablets** would be required for a 7 day course.

(iii) Body weight of animal = 280 kg
Tablets given per day (24 hr period) = **4 tablets**

Daily dose of drug $= 560$ mg (given in question)

(a) Tablet strength $= \dfrac{560\,\text{mg}}{4\,\text{tablets}} = \mathbf{140\ mg/tablet}$

(b) Dose rate is weight of drug administered in 24 hr period/body weight

$= \dfrac{560\,\text{mg}}{280\,\text{kg}} = \mathbf{2\ mg/kg/day}$

(c) Total weight of drug $= 7$ days $\times 560$ mg

$\qquad\qquad\qquad\qquad = 3920$ mg $= \mathbf{3.92\,g}$

(iv) Body weight of hamster $= 125$ g

Dose rate $= 1$ mg/kg/8 hrs

Drug requirement per dose $= \dfrac{1\,\text{mg} \times 125\,\text{g}}{1000}$

(hamster's weight of 125 g is divided by 1000 to convert it to kg)

$\qquad\qquad\qquad = 0.125$ mg of drug per dose

Doses per day $= \dfrac{24\,\text{hrs}}{8\,\text{hrs}}$

$\qquad\quad = 3$ doses each requiring 0.125 mg

$\qquad\quad = 3 \times 0.125$ mg $= 0.375$ mg/day

Strength of suspension $= 0.25$ mg/ml

Therefore daily requirement $= \dfrac{0.375\,\text{mg}}{0.25\,\text{mg}}$

$\qquad\qquad\qquad\qquad = 1.5$ ml per day for 7 days

$\qquad$ 7 day course $= \mathbf{10.5\ ml}$

(v) Body weight of kitten $= 1$ kg

Dosage rate 60 mg/kg/day $= 60$ mg

Total drug intake recommended $= 0.3$ g

$\qquad\qquad\qquad\qquad\qquad = (0.3 \times 1000)$ mg

$\qquad\qquad\qquad\qquad\qquad = 300$ mg

To find the number of tablets $= \dfrac{300\,\text{mg}}{30\,\text{mg}}$ tablet $= 10$ tablets.

8 tablets have already been administered over the last 4 days (i.e. 1 b.i.d.)

One more day will complete the prescribed course.

(vi) Body weight of bird is $33\,lb = 15\,kg$
Amount of drug taken over 1 day
$= 2 \times 12.5\,mg$ b.i.d. i.e. $25\,mg$ b.i.d.
$= 50\,mg/day$

$$\textbf{Dose rate} = \frac{\textbf{daily weight of drug in mg}}{\textbf{body weight of patient in kg}}$$

For the bird weighing $15\,kg$, the dose rate would be $\dfrac{50\,mg}{15\,kg}$

$= \textbf{3.33\,mg/kg/day}$
For a bird weighing $44\,lb$ ($20\,kg$), the total dose in 5 days
$= (3.33\,mg \times 20\,kg)$ per day $\times$ 5 days
$= 66.6\,mg$ per day $\times$ 5 days
$= \textbf{333\,mg total dose}$

(vii) Body weight of dog $= 5\,kg$
Dose rate $= 4\,mg/kg/day$
Dose $= 4\,mg \times 5\,kg/day$
$\qquad = 20\,mg/day$
Tablets contain $2.5\,mg$ of the drug therefore
number of tablets required per day $= \dfrac{20\,mg}{2.5\,mg} = 8$ tablets
Therefore **4 tablets** should be given b.i.d.

(viii) Body weight of kitten $= \dfrac{1500\,g}{1000} = 1.5\,kg$

($1500\,g$ is divided by 1000 to change g into kg)
Required amount of drug per day $= 12\,mg \times 2$
$\qquad\qquad\qquad\qquad\qquad\quad = 24\,mg/day$
The kitten needs $\dfrac{24\,mg}{1.5\,kg}$
Therefore dose rate $= \textbf{16\,mg/kg/day}$

Note that tablet strength is irrelevant to the calculation and is not required as part of the final answer, as only the dose rate is required. Questions such as this, which may contain unnecessary additional information, could arise in examinations.

(ix) Total amount of drug administered daily to the animal
    = 2 tablets × 15 mg = 30 mg every 8 hrs
                = 90 mg per day
        Dose rate = 5 mg/kg/day
    To find the weight of the animal
    $$\frac{90\,\text{mg/day}}{5\,\text{mg/kg/day}} = \textbf{18 kg (answer c)}$$

(x) Weight of antibiotic per ml = 5 mg
    Number of ml administered every 6 hrs = 4 ml
    Weight of antibiotic ingested every 6 hrs = 5 mg × 4 ml
                    = 20 mg
    Weight of antibiotic ingested every 24 hrs
    = 20 mg q.i.d. = 80 mg
    $$\text{Dose rate} = \frac{80\,\text{mg/day}}{50\,\text{kg}} = \textbf{1.6 mg/kg/day}$$

Chapter 6

Dosages – Injections

These extremely important calculations usually relate a drug dosage to an animal's body weight and the period of time over which it has to be administered. Thus, the dose rate is normally expressed in the units mg/kg/day; that is, milligrams per kilogram of the drug to be given, multiplied by the animal's body weight in kilograms, to be administered over a given time period.

There is always a time element involved such as twice daily (b.i.d.). It may be that the weight is given in lb rather than kg. The conversion from lb to kg is a fairly easy conversion. This is because 1 kg converts to 2.2 lb (approximately). Therefore:

$10 \text{ kg} = 22 \text{ lb}$
$15 \text{ kg} = 33 \text{ lb}$
$20 \text{ kg} = 44 \text{ lb}$
$25 \text{ kg} = 55 \text{ lb}$
$30 \text{ kg} = 66 \text{ lb}$

Example 1

Calculate the volume of drug required to treat a bird weighing 15 g if the dose rate is 200 μg/kg body weight.

Answer

First the body weight must be converted to kg:

$$15g = \frac{15}{1000} \text{ kg} = 0.015 \text{ kg}$$

Next multiply the body weight by the dose rate.

Therefore dose $= 0.015\,\text{kg} \times 200\,\mu\text{g} = \mathbf{3\mu g}$

Example 2

A 33 lb dog has to be treated with a drug at a dose rate of $10\,\mu\text{g/kg}$. Calculate the amount of drug required.

Answer

First convert the dog's weight to kg by dividing by 2.2 or by multiplying by 0.45 (see conversion factors in Chapter 1).

$$33\,\text{lb} = \frac{33}{2.2}\,\text{kg} = 15\,\text{kg}$$

Next multiply the weight in kg by the dose rate.

Therefore, dose $= 15\,\text{kg} \times 10\,\mu\text{g} = \mathbf{150\,\mu g}$

Example 3

The drug used to treat the dog in example 2 is in the form of a 0.02% solution. Calculate what volume of the solution will be required.

Answer

First convert $150\,\mu\text{g}$ to g by dividing by one million (move decimal point 6 places to the left).

Therefore $150\mu\text{g} = 0.00015\,\text{g}$

Next change the standard formula for a % solution as shown below

$$\% \text{ solution} = \frac{\text{weight in g}}{\text{volume in ml}} \times 100$$

$$\text{Therefore volume in ml} = \frac{\text{weight in g}}{\% \text{ solution}} \times 100$$

$$= \frac{0.00015\,g \times 100}{0.02} = \frac{0.015}{0.02}$$

$$= \mathbf{0.75\,ml}$$

Note that dividing 0.015 by 0.02 is the same as dividing 1.5 by 2 which is a more simple calculation!

Self-test exercise
(fully-worked answers at the end of this chapter)

(i)   A dog weighing 66 lb needs to be treated with a drug at a dose rate of 5 mg/kg/day.
The solution available is 2%.
Calculate the volume in ml of the daily injection to give the correct dose.

(ii)   A 2.5 kg Chihuahua needs two × 5 ml injections daily of a 0.3% solution of a drug.
Calculate the dose rate in mg/kg/day.

(iii)   A Toucan requires a daily injection of 0.06 g of a drug which is contained in a 10% solution.
Calculate the dose rate if the Toucan weighs 1.5 kg.

(iv)   5 ml of a 0.03% solution of a drug is administered to a 200 g toad.
Calculate the dosage administered.

(v)   A kitten is given an injection of a 0.5% solution.
The dose rate is 1 mg/kg/day and the kitten weighs 0.5 kg.
Calculate what volume is injected.

(vi)   A python weighing 70 kg needs an injection. The recommended dose rate of the prescribed drug is 2 mg/kg/day.

If the python has two injections/day, what volume is required for each injection of the 2% solution in which the drug is available?

(vii)　A guinea pig has to be treated with a drug at a dose rate of 20 mg/kg/8 hrs.

It weighs 750 g and the drug is only available as a 2.5% solution.

What is the volume of each injection?

Would this change if the weight of the guinea pig was 1.5 kg and the solution's concentration increased to 5%?

(viii)　A gerbil needs a 0.5 ml injection of a 2% solution over a 24 hour period.

What is the dose rate if the gerbil weighs 60 g.

(ix)　A 7.5 kg dog needs two daily injections.

If each injection is 15 ml, calculate the dose rate in mg/kg/day.

What weight of the drug, in g, will be administered over a 5 day period if the solution used is of 2.5% concentration.

(x)　A dog weighing 8 kg needs injections t.i.d. of a 4% solution.

Calculate the weight in mg of the drug and the volume in ml that it receives per injection.

Assume a dose rate of 6 mg/kg/8 hrs.

Answers to self-test exercise

(i)　Weight of dog $= 66\,lb = \dfrac{66}{2.2} = 30\,kg$

Dosage 5 mg/kg/day $= 5\,mg/kg \times 30\,kg$

$\qquad\qquad\qquad\quad = 150\,mg$

$\qquad\qquad\qquad\quad = \dfrac{150\,mg}{1000} = 0.15\,g$

Solution available　$= 2\,\%$

To solve this problem, the volume of 2% solution that is required contains 0.15 g of the drug.

Using the formula for the percentage solution (from Chapter 3),

$$\% \text{ solution} = \frac{\text{weight in g}}{\text{volume in ml}} \times 100$$

The % solution and weight in g is either given or can be calculated from the data presented.

From this and by manipulating the formula above, the volume can be calculated:

$$\text{volume in ml} = \frac{\text{weight in g}}{\% \text{ solution}} \times 100$$

(See Chapter 3 to understand how the formula was manipulated.)

Substituting the values into the formula gives:

$$\text{volume in ml} = \frac{0.15 \,\text{g} \times 100}{2\%} = \textbf{7.5 ml}$$

(ii) Using the formula

$$\% \text{ solution} = \frac{\text{weight in g}}{\text{volume in ml}} \times 100$$

$$\text{Therefore weight in g} = \frac{\% \text{ solution} \times \text{volume in ml}}{100}$$

2 daily injections of 5 ml are given i.e. 10 ml/day
Substituting values into the formula gives the following

$$\text{weight in g} = \frac{0.3\% \times 10 \,\text{ml}}{100}$$

$$= \frac{3}{100}$$

$$= 0.03 \,\text{g per day}$$

$$= 30 \,\text{mg/day}$$

Dose rate is therefore 30 mg/day/2.5 kg of body weight. This can be expressed as a dose rate of **12 mg/kg/day**.

(iii)   Sometimes, non-essential information is included in an exam question! Notice that the % value of the solution is immaterial as the question states that the solution contains 0.06 g of drug.

As the body weight has already been given as 1.5 kg, the dose can be calculated from these two pieces of data i.e. the dosage rate can be calculated by dividing 0.06 g by the bird's weight.

$$\text{i.e. } 0.06\,\text{g} \times \frac{1000}{1.5} = \textbf{40 mg /kg /day}$$

NB Multiplying by 1000 converts g to mg and the dosage can be expressed in the conventional way in mg/kg/day.

(iv)   Using the usual formula with the correct units, the given quantities can be substituted into the formula.

$$0.03\% \text{ solution} = \frac{\text{weight in g}}{5\,\text{ml}} \times 100$$

Rearranging the formula to make the unknown value (in this case the weight in g) the subject of the equation gives

$$\begin{aligned}
\text{weight} &= \frac{0.03\%}{100} \times 5\,\text{ml} \\
&= 0.0015\,\text{g} \\
&= 0.0015 \times 1000\,\text{mg} \\
&= 1.5\,\text{mg}
\end{aligned}$$

Toad weighs $\dfrac{200\,\text{g}}{1000} = 0.2\,\text{kg}$

Therefore dose rate is 1.5 mg/0.2 kg/day

Note that the mg need to be expressed per kg, therefore the 0.2 kg must be multiplied by 5 to get to 1 kg, hence the 1.5 mg also needs to be multiplied by 5 to keep the ratios consistent.

Therefore the dose rate is **7.5 mg/kg/day**

(v) Dosage rate is given as 1 mg/kg/day
The kitten weighs 0.5 kg therefore using the above dosage it only requires 0.5 mg of the sedative per day.
The drug is available in a 0.5% solution.
The answer to the question lies in the calculation of the volume which contains 0.5 mg of the drug.
This can be achieved by using the standard formula

$$\% \text{ solution} = \frac{\text{weight in g}}{\text{volume in ml}} \times 100$$

As the question has given two of the elements (% solution and weight) of this formula, the missing element (volume) is the answer to the question. Substituting the given figures in the correct units gives:

$$0.5\% = \frac{(0.5\,\text{g}/1000)}{\text{volume in ml}} \times 100$$

$$\left(\text{note } 0.5\,\text{mg} = \frac{0.5}{1000}\,\text{g}\right)$$

Rearranging the formula and calculating the units gives the following:

$$\text{volume in ml} = \frac{0.0005\,\text{g}}{0.5\%} \times 100 = \mathbf{0.1\,ml}$$

(vi) Python's body weight = 70 kg
Dose = 2 mg/kg/day
Weight required to be administered per day is
2 mg × 70 kg = 140 mg
i.e 70 mg or 0.07 g per injection, twice a day (stated in question)
Using the standard formula

$$\% \text{ solution} = \frac{\text{weight in g}}{\text{volume in ml}} \times 100$$

Substituting known values

$$2\% = \frac{0.07\,\text{g}}{\text{volume in ml}} \times 100$$

$$\text{volume in ml} = \frac{0.07\,\text{g}}{2\%} \times 100$$

$$= 3.5\,\text{ml}$$

(vii)   Body weight of guinea pig $= 750\,\text{g} = 0.75\,\text{kg}$
Dose rate $= 20\,\text{mg/kg/8 hrs}$
Notice that the guinea pig weighs **less** than 1 kg!
Weight of drug required for this guinea pig is
$20\,\text{mg} \times$ body weight $(0.75\,\text{kg}) = 15\,\text{mg}$ every 8 hrs
Therefore weight of each injection is $15\,\text{mg} = 0.015\,\text{g}$
Using the standard formula

$$\% \text{ solution} = \frac{\text{weight in g}}{\text{volume in ml}} \times 100$$

Substituting the given values gives

$$2.5\% = (0.015\,\text{g/volume in ml}) \times 100$$

$$\text{volume in ml} = \frac{0.015\,\text{g} \times 100}{2.5\%}$$

$$= \textbf{0.6 ml per injection}$$

If the weight of the guinea pig were doubled to 1.5 kg and the dosage rate remained the same, the guinea pig would require twice as much weight of drug per injection i.e. $20\,\text{mg} \times$ body weight $(1.5\,\text{kg})$
$= 30\,\text{mg}$ every 8 hrs
If the solution available were now a 5% solution, the standard formula above would give the following figures

$$5\% = \frac{0.030\,\text{g}}{\text{volume in ml}} \times 100$$

$$\text{volume in ml} = \frac{0.030\,\text{g}}{5\%} \times 100 = \textbf{0.6 ml per injection}$$

Therefore, the volume would remain the same but the concentration would have doubled.

(viii)   Body weight of gerbil = 60 g
Period of administration = 24 hrs
Solution strength = 2%
Volume of solution used = 0.5 ml
The question asks for the dose rate to be calculated.
The missing piece of data is the weight injected into the gerbil contained in the 0.5 ml of 2% solution.
Standard formula is

$$\% \text{ solution} = \frac{\text{weight in g}}{\text{volume in ml}} \times 100$$

This can be rearranged to give

$$\text{weight in g} = \frac{\% \text{ solution} \times \text{volume in ml}}{100}$$

$$\text{weight in g} = \frac{2\% \times 0.5 \, \text{ml}}{100} = 0.01 \, \text{g}$$

0.01 g converts to 10 mg (1000 × 0.01 mg = 10 mg)

$$\text{Dose rate} = \frac{10 \, \text{mg/day}}{60 \, \text{g}}$$

This ratio must to be converted to mg/kg/day, i.e. the bottom figure of 60 g must be 'factored up' to 1 kg and the 'factor' required to do this must then be used on the top figure to keep the dose rate in proportion. This will then convert the dose rate above into the units required in the question.
To 'factor up' 60 g to 1 kg, divide by 60 and multiply by 1000.
The same must be done for the top figure of 10 mg

$$\frac{10 \, \text{mg}}{60} \times 1000 = \textbf{166.7} \, \text{mg/day}$$

The dose rate would be expressed as **166.7 mg/kg/day**

(ix)   Body weight of dog $= 7.5$ kg
Period of administration $= 12$ hours
Volume of solution administered $= 2 \times 15$ ml $= 30$ ml
Solution strength $= 2.5\%$
The question asks for the dose rate to be calculated in mg/kg/day.
The best approach to this question is to calculate the weight of drug which is injected into the dog, contained in the daily administered volume.
This is two injections of 15 ml every day $= 30$ ml/day.
This is done by applying the standard formula for a % solution and substituting the known values.

$$\% \text{ solution} = \frac{\text{weight in g}}{\text{volume in ml}} \times 100$$

Therefore weight in g $= \%$ solution $\times \dfrac{\text{volume in ml}}{100}$

Substituting known values gives

$$\text{weight in g} = \frac{2.5\% \text{ solution} \times 30 \text{ ml}}{100}$$

weight in g $= 0.75$ g administered every day

To convert this weight into mg (required to give the answer in the required units), multiply by 1000.

Weight in mg $= 0.75$ g $\times 1000 = 750$ mg/day

Expressing this in terms of the body weight of the dog

$$\frac{750 \text{ mg}}{7.5 \text{ kg}} = \mathbf{100 \, mg/kg/day.}$$

The question also asks for the weight in g administered over 5 days.
This quantity was calculated earlier in the answer as 0.75 g/day.
The amount of drug administered over a 5 day period is 5×0.75 g $= \mathbf{3.75 \, g}$

(x)   Body weight of dog $= 8.0$ kg
Dose rate $= 6$ mg/kg/8 hrs
Solution strength $= 4\%$
Weight of drug required $=$ body weight $\times$ dose rate
Substitute known values $= 8$ kg $\times$ 6 mg/kg/8 hrs
$= $ **48 mg every 8 hrs** (per injection)
Standard formula for % solution is

$$\% \text{ solution} = \frac{\text{weight in g}}{\text{volume in ml}} \times 100$$

In this formula the weight and the % concentration are known.
The volume is to be calculated

$$\text{volume in ml} = \frac{\text{weight in g}}{\% \text{ solution}} \times 100$$

(See chapter on percentage solutions (Chapter 3) to understand how the formula was manipulated.)

$$\text{volume in ml} = \frac{0.048 \text{ g}}{4\% \text{ solution}} \times 100$$
$$= \textbf{1.2 ml} \text{ per injection}$$

Chapter 7

Rehydration of the Patient

There are various ways of estimating the fluid replacement needs of an animal, some of which are more accurate than others. When replacing fluids by infusion it is important to replace the:

- existing fluid deficit
- maintenance needs
- any ongoing losses

This chapter looks at the ways in which fluid deficit is estimated, for example by:

- assuming that fluid maintenance volumes are about the same per kg for all species and individuals
- using the clinical history given by an animal's owner
- noting the clinical (cardinal) symptoms and using a chart (see later) to assess the percentage dehydration

There are also ways in which fluid deficit and replacement needs are further estimated by carrying out a calculation to achieve a reasonable approximate deficit for rehydration purposes, for example by:

- multiplying the assessed % dehydration by the body weight in kg
- carrying out a packed cell volume (PCV) and using the % increase above the average normal value for each species to calculate the amount of fluid deficit

Replacement of normal daily fluid loss

Although a daily fluid loss, i.e. a deficit, will vary between species and individuals, it is now widely accepted that an average replacement or maintenance volume is 50 ml/kg/24 hrs. This is based on:

insensible losses	$= 20$ ml/kg/day
(respiration and sweating)	
urine	$= 20$ ml/kg/day
faeces	$= 10$ ml/kg/day
total losses	$= \mathbf{50}$ **ml/kg/day**

Under normal circumstances, animals will replace this deficit with fluid taken in by drinking and eating and adjusting this intake when the deficit increases, e.g. after exercise.

However, when carrying out calculations related to fluid therapy requirements, the replacement of normal daily losses are usually included and are referred to as the maintenance requirement.

Assessment of % dehydration based on clinical history

This is the least accurate method of assessing % dehydration as it relies on obtaining a reasonable clinical history from an animal's owner, such as how many times a day the animal has vomited and encouraging the owner to estimate the volume produced on each occasion.

It is unlikely that many owners will relate volume of fluid lost to millilitres, but they should be able to relate it to typical household measurements, with which they are familiar.

However, it is important to recognise that this is only a guide and cannot be relied upon to give a very accurate estimate of the fluid deficit. The calculated amount of fluid lost is based on the 'anecdotal' evidence of an owner who may not be a very observant or objective witness.

Example 1

A dog weighing 15 kg has been vomiting 5 times a day for 3 days and is presented at evening surgery. The owner states that:

'the dog has been vomiting for the last 3 days, about 5 times a day, producing about a tablespoonful each time'.

What is the total volume of fluid lost in the vomit?

Answer

In this instance, the weight of 15 kg is irrelevant and the fluid deficit is based only on the owner's perception of the situation.

1 tablespoon (standard) is equivalent to 15 ml (see Chapter 1 for conversion of household measurements)

5×15 ml $= 75$ ml of fluid lost in vomit/day
3 days $\times 75$ ml $= \textbf{225 ml}$ total fluid deficit lost in the vomit

Assessment of % dehydration based on weight

When an animal is presented at the surgery with such a history, a far more accurate method of estimating the amount of fluid lost in the vomit, is to base it on the animal's weight.

It is usual to assume that diarrhoea and vomit are lost at a rate of 4 ml/kg/day of body weight.

Example 2

A dog weighing 15 kg which has vomited 5 times a day for 3 days is presented at evening surgery. Assume that vomit is lost at the rate of 4 ml/kg/day. What is the total volume of fluid lost in the vomit?

Answer

15 kg × 4 ml = 60 ml
5 × 60 ml = 300 ml
3 days × 300 ml = **900 ml** total fluid deficit lost in the vomit

Assessment of % dehydration based on laboratory diagnosis

Fluid deficit can be assessed by carrying out a packed cell volume (PCV) and assuming that every 1% increase is equivalent to a 10 ml/kg deficit. Unless the normal value for an individual patient has been recorded beforehand, the % increase has to be taken as being above the average normal values for each species, such as:

normal average PCV value = 45% for a dog
= 35% for a cat

Example 3

A dog weighing 15 kg has been vomiting 5 times a day for 3 days and is presented at evening surgery. A PCV is carried out and gives a reading of 52%. What is the total volume of fluid lost in the vomit?

Answer

PCV reading = 52%
Normal PCV (dog) = 45%
(52% − 45%) = 7% increase from the normal average
7 × 10 ml = 70 ml
15 kg dog × 70 ml = **1050 ml** total fluid deficit lost in the vomit

Note

- As PCV will decrease in cases of anaemia or acute blood loss, this method of fluid deficit assessment should *not* be used for such patients.

Assessment of % dehydration based on clinical symptoms

Clinical symptoms can be used to assess percentage dehydration. See table 7.1.

Once a visual assessment of % dehydration has been made using the clinical symptoms, a calculation based on this and the weight of the animal can then be carried out to estimate the fluid deficit which needs to be replaced.

Table 7.1 Assessment of percentage dehydration

Clinical symptoms	Estimated % dehydration
Urine looks and smells more concentrated	Less than 5%
Some loss of elasticity to skin	Approximately 6% (range 5–6%)
No skin elasticity 'Sticky' mucous membranes Eyes softening/slight sunken appearance Capillary refill time (CRT) slightly above the normal of 2 seconds	Approximately 7% (range 6–8%)
Skin is easily 'tented' and stays in place when pinched 'Sticky' mucous membranes Eyes obviously sunken CRT obviously prolonged Low urine output (oliguria)	Approximately 11% (range 10–12%)
Shock Death impending	Approximately 14% (range 12–15%)

Example 4

A dog weighing 15 kg has been vomiting 5 times a day for 3 days and is presented at evening surgery. It is showing clinical symptoms typical of about 7% dehydration. What is the total volume of fluid lost in the vomit?

Answer

Using the formula:

body weight (kg) × % dehydration (changed into a decimal)
= 15 × 0.07 = 1.05 litres (×1000 to find number of ml)
= **1050 ml** total fluid deficit

or alternatively use the quicker formula

body weight (kg) × % dehydration × 10
= 15 × 7 × 10 = **1050 ml** total fluid deficit

It can be seen that estimating fluid deficit using the anecdotal clinical history in example 1, is the most inaccurate. The total volume calculated in example 1 is vastly different when compared to the totals calculated in examples 2, 3 and 4.

Calculation of total fluid requirements

It should be noted from the beginning of the chapter that, when replacing fluids by infusion, it is important to replace the:

- existing fluid deficit
- maintenance needs
- any ongoing losses

and a calculation can be carried out to include all of these requirements.

Example 5

A dog weighing 15 kg has been vomiting 5 times a day for 3 days and is presented at evening surgery. It is showing clinical symptoms typical of 7% dehydration. Calculate the total fluid replacement requirement over the next 24 hrs for this animal.

> Body weight (kg) × % dehydration × 10
> $= 15 \times 7 \times 10 = 1050$ ml total fluid deficit
> Body weight (kg) × maintenance requirements per 24 hrs
> $= 15 \times 50 = 750$ ml total maintenance requirements
> Body weight (kg) × ongoing losses per 24 hrs taken as 4 ml/kg vomit, in this case vomiting 5 times in 24 hrs.
> $= 15 \times 4 = 60$ ml × 5 times/24 hrs
> $\qquad = 300$ ml total ongoing losses
> Adding together the total fluid deficit, maintenance requirement and the ongoing losses to find the total fluid requirement over 24 hrs, gives
> total fluid requirement $= \mathbf{2100\ ml\ over\ 24\ hrs}$

It will sometimes be necessary to replace the total deficit more quickly than over 24 hrs and, if this is the case, a proportion of the daily maintenance requirements should also be given during this shorter period.

Example 6

A dog weighing 15 kg has been vomiting 5 times a day for 3 days and is presented at evening surgery. It is showing clinical symptoms typical of 7% dehydration.

(a)   Calculate the total fluid replacement requirement over the next 24 hrs, for this animal.
(b)   The veterinary surgeon requires the total deficit plus a proportional amount of the daily total fluid maintenance to be given over the first 8 hrs. Calculate this amount.

Answer

It can be seen from example 5 that:

(a) 1050 ml = total fluid deficit

    750 ml = total maintenance requirements

    Total fluid replacement requirement = **1800 ml over next 24 hrs**

    Ongoing losses are not mentioned in this question and therefore cannot be included in the total amount.

(b) To find the fluid which must be given in 8 hrs:

$$\frac{24\,\text{hrs}}{8\,\text{hrs}} = 3 \text{ (i.e. in } \tfrac{1}{3} \text{ of 24 hrs)}$$

Total maintenance per 24 hrs is 750 ml; divide this amount by 3:

$$\frac{750\text{ml}}{3} = 250\,\text{ml total maintenance in 8 hrs}$$

The dog needs 250 ml maintenance fluid, plus the total fluid deficit over the next 8 hrs. Therefore add these two totals together:

250 ml + 1050 ml = **1300 ml over the next 8 hrs**

Note

It is very important to remember the following points when calculating the infused fluid requirements of an animal.

- Obese animals should have all fluid replacement calculated on estimated 'normal' body weight. This is because fat cells hold less water, but take up more room, than other tissue cells. It would therefore be possible to over-hydrate an obese patient and cause pulmonary oedema, which can be fatal.
- Where colloid (as opposed to crystalloid) infusions are to be given, manufacturers' instructions should always be checked carefully to ascertain if there is a limit to the amount of ml which can be administered safely per kg over a particular time period, e.g. over 24 hours. The remainder of the deficit is usually made up by infusing with a crystalloid.

- Once the total amount of fluid replacement to be given over a certain time period, e.g. 24 hours, has been estimated, it will then be necessary to work out the drip rate. For these calculations see Chapter 8 (Fluid Therapy – Rates of Administration).

Self-test exercise
(fully-worked answers at the end of this chapter)

(i)   A 3 kg Pomeranian dog is brought into the surgery showing 5% dehydration. Calculate the fluid it needs to receive over 24 hours, for both maintenance and deficit requirements.

(ii) A 22 lb Dachshund has had acute vomiting and diarrhoea, vomiting 6 times and producing diarrhoea 5 times, within the last 24 hours. What is the total fluid deficit?

(iii) A 20 kg cross-bred Collie bitch needs a hysterectomy due to a closed pyometra. She is very toxic and weak, having vomited 7 times in the last 24 hours. She is still vomiting at the same rate and the veterinary surgeon prescribes rehydration for 2 hours prior to surgery to improve the prognosis. The PCV reading is 56%. Infusion will continue throughout and following surgery, and fluid replacement calculations will need to be carried out daily. Calculate the fluid deficit, ongoing losses and maintenance requirements for the bitch over the initial 24 hour period.

(iv) A 9 kg Tibetan terrier is brought in with arterial haemorrhaging, following a road traffic accident (RTA). The haemorrhaging is arrested by the veterinary team and the dog is to be infused, rather than transfused as there is no whole blood available. The dog is showing clinical symptoms typical of 10% dehydration, although a PCV gives a reading of 51%. Calculate the fluid replacement requirement for this dog over the next 24 hours.

(v)   A 5 kg New Zealand white rabbit has been off its food and water for four days due to malocclusion. It is showing clinical symptoms typical of about 8% dehydration. Calculate the fluid requirement for the next 24 hour period.

(vi)   A stray cat weighing 2.2 kg is brought in suffering from malnutrition. It is showing clinical symptoms of pale mucous membranes and there is some loss of elasticity to its skin. Blood is taken for laboratory diagnosis and a blood smear with Giemsa's stain and a PCV are carried out. The blood parasite, *Haemobartonella felis* is confirmed and the PCV reading is 43%. Calculate the fluid deficit and ongoing maintenance requirements for fluid replacement over the next 24 hour period.

(vii) Following open reduction of a fractured femur, a 5.5 kg Manchester terrier has become anorexic and has refused to drink for 24 hours. Its urine is very concentrated and smelly, but the animal shows no other signs of dehydration. As it will still not be persuaded to eat or drink, and its PCV has a reading of 50%, it will be necessary to carry out fluid therapy. Calculate the fluid replacement requirements for this dog over the next 24 hours.

(viii) Following a poor hibernation, a dehydrated and anorexic tortoise needs to be properly rehydrated before it has food administered. This is in order to make sure the intestinal villi are standing up and able to absorb food. This rehydration will take at least 2 weeks of daily stomach tubing before food supplements can safely be tubed, otherwise diarrhoea will occur causing further dehydration and the reptile is still likely to die. The tortoise weighs 2400 g. As the metabolic rate of reptiles is very slow when compared to the mammal, it will be rehydrated by replacing the fluid at the normal maintenance rate of 50 ml/kg of body weight/day. This is to be given by stomach tube.

    (a) Calculate the amount of fluid needed per day.

    (b) As a tortoise of this size and in this condition would have a stomach capacity of about 20 ml, how many times a day would this tortoise need to be stomach tubed during that time period?

    (c) To both fit in with the working day and allow the tortoise to rest at night, the total amount would need to be administered over 12 hours – how often would the tortoise need to be stomach tubed?

(ix)   Following the ingestion of a cooked bone, a Dalmation dog has vomited 9 times over 36 hours prior to being presented at surgery. Prior to being anaesthetised, the dog was weighed and found to be 29 kg, i.e. about 6 kg overweight. An enterotomy was necessary and the veterinary surgeon prescribed nil by mouth for 24 hours. Calculate the fluid deficit, plus the maintenance requirements for this dog for the next 24 hours.

(x)   A hedgehog is presented with an open wound which is infested with maggots; the animal is in toxic shock as a result. It is weighed before it is anaesthetised, and is found to be underweight at 0.9 kg. The maggots are removed, but it is showing all the clinical symptoms of 12% dehydration.

    (a) Calculate the fluid deficit and the maintenance replacement requirements for the next 24 hours.

    (b) The veterinary surgeon wants the full fluid deficit, plus the fluid maintenance requirements for 6 hours, to be given over the next 6 hours. Calculate what this amount will be.

Answers to self-test exercise

(i)   A 3 kg Pomeranian, showing 5% dehydration needs 24 hrs of fluid therapy for both maintenance and deficit.

To find the deficit, use the formula:

Body weight (kg) × % dehydration × 10
3 kg × 5% × 10 = 150 ml = total fluid deficit

To find the maintenance requirements:

Body weight (kg) × maintenance requirements per 24 hrs
3 kg × 50 ml = 150 ml = total maintenance requirements
Total fluid requirement: **300 ml over 24 hrs**

(ii) A 22 lb Dachshund with acute vomiting and diarrhoea for 24 hours. Calculate the *fluid deficit* (only this is asked for here).

First convert lb (pounds) to kg by dividing 22 lb by 2.2
$$\frac{22\,lb}{2.2} = 10\,kg$$

Assume 4 ml is lost per kg in *both* the diarrhoea and vomiting.

10 kg × 4 ml = 40 ml
Vomiting: 6 × 40 ml = 240 ml
Diarrhoea: 5 × 40 ml = 200 ml
Total = **480 ml total fluid deficit**

(iii) A 20 kg cross-bred Collie bitch needs a hysterectomy due to a closed pyometra. She needs rehydration for 3 hours prior to the surgery. Her PCV reading is 56%. Calculate the fluid deficit and maintenance requirements over the initial 24 hour period.

The 2 hour pre-operative infusion is irrelevant to this calculation, but the question requires the fluid deficit and maintenance requirements to be calculated over the initial 24 hour period.

As there is a PCV reading which can be used, the losses from vomiting during the previous 24 hr period do not have to be calculated separately.

PCV reading of 56% (56%–45%) = an increase of 11%
Each 1% increase represents 10 ml deficit:

11×10 ml $= 110$ ml
20 kg $\times 110$ ml $= 2200$ ml total fluid deficit

Vomiting is still occurring and it must be assumed that ongoing losses will continue at the same rate, i.e. 4 ml/kg of body weight, 7 times a day:

20 kg $\times 4$ ml $= 80$ ml
7 times in 24 hrs $= 560$ ml total ongoing losses

Normal maintenance rates need to be included, as 50 ml/kg/24 hrs

20 kg $\times 50$ ml $= 1000$ ml total maintenance needs
Total fluid requirement $= \textbf{3760 ml in 24 hrs}$

(iv) A 9 kg Tibetan terrier, suffering from arterial haemorrhaging following an RTA. The haemorrhaging has been arrested, but the dog is showing clinical symptoms typical of 10% dehydration, although a PCV reading is 51%, i.e. 6% above the normal for a dog of 45%.

The fluid requirements need to be calculated over the next 24 hrs. As the dog has been haemorrhaging, the PCV reading should not be used here: the clinical symptoms which indicate 10% dehydration should be taken. To find the deficit use the formula:

body weight (kg) $\times$ % dehydration $\times 10$
$9 \times 10 \times 10 = 900$ ml total fluid deficit

To find the normal fluid maintenance of 50 ml/kg/24 hrs:

9 kg $\times 50$ ml $= 450$ ml total maintenance needs

There are no ongoing losses to include, therefore:

Total fluid requirement $= \textbf{1350 ml in 24 hrs}$

(v) A 5 kg rabbit off food and water for four days, with clinical symptoms typical of 8% dehydration. Calculate the fluid required for the next 24 hrs.
To find the deficit, use the formula:

$$5 \text{ kg} \times 8\% \times 10 = 400 \text{ ml total fluid deficit}$$

To find the normal fluid maintenance of 50 ml/kg/24 hrs:

$$5 \text{ kg} \times 50 \text{ ml} = 250 \text{ ml total maintenance needs}$$
Total fluid requirement = **650 ml in 24 hrs**

(vi) A stray cat suffering from malnutrition and weighing only 2.2 kg. It has pale mucous membranes and the Giemsa's blood smear is positive for *H. felis*, which indicates anaemia.

The PCV is 43%, i.e. 8% above the normal average for the cat (35%). However, there is some loss of elasticity to its skin, which from Table 7.1 indicates dehydration to be about 6%. As this cat is anaemic, the PCV reading for this cat should not be used. Therefore to find the fluid deficit use the 6% figure, with the formula:

$$2.2 \text{ kg} \times 6\% \times 10 = 132 \text{ ml total fluid deficit}$$

To find the normal fluid maintenance of 50 ml/kg/24 hrs:

$$2.2 \text{ kg} \times 50 \text{ ml} = 110 \text{ ml total maintenance needs}$$
Total fluid requirement = **242 ml in 24 hrs**

(vii) A 5.5 kg Manchester terrier has been anorexic and refused to drink for 24 hrs, with the result that its urine has become very concentrated and smelly. The PCV has a reading of 50%, i.e. (50%–45%) = 5% above the normal average for a dog. Calculate the fluid replacement requirements over the next 24 hrs. To find the deficit, use the formula:

$$5.5 \text{ kg} \times 5\% \times 10 = 275 \text{ ml total fluid deficit}$$

To find the normal fluid maintenance of 50 ml/kg/24 hrs:

5.5 kg × 50 ml = 275 ml total maintenance needs
Total fluid requirement = **550 ml in 24 hrs**

(viii) A tortoise weighs 2400 g and needs 50 ml/kg body weight/day. To find the weight in kg, divide 2400 g by 1000 (as there are 1000 g in 1 kg):

$$\frac{2400\,g}{1000} = 2.4\,kg$$

(a) To find how many ml are needed per day by the tortoise:

2.4 kg × 50 ml = 120 ml

Total fluid requirement = 120 ml per day.

(b) This tortoise has a stomach capacity of about 20 ml. The number of times per day the tortoise is stomach tubed is:

$$\frac{120\,ml}{20\,ml} = \textbf{6 times per day}$$

(c) To find how often the tortoise needs to be stomach tubed over 12 hrs:

$$\frac{12\,hrs}{6\ \text{times per day}} = \textbf{every 2 hrs}$$

The tortoise needs to be stomach tubed **every 2 hrs**.

(ix) A 29 kg Dalmation has vomited 9 times over 36 hrs. Calculate the fluid requirements for the next 24 hrs.
To find the fluid deficit, assume vomit is lost at the rate of 4 ml/kg body weight, using the normal body weight (23 kg) in the formula.

23 kg × 4 ml = 92 ml

Vomited: 9×92 ml $= 828$ ml total fluid deficit

To find the normal fluid maintenance of 50 ml/kg/24 hrs:

23 kg $\times 50$ ml $= 1150$ ml total maintenance needs
Total fluid requirement $= $ **1978 ml in 24 hrs**

(x) A hedgehog weighing 0.9 kg is in toxic shock with clinical symptoms typical of 12% dehydration.

(a) Calculate the fluid deficit and the maintenance replacement requirements for the next 24 hrs.
To find the deficit, use the formula:

0.9 kg $\times 12\% \times 10 = 108$ ml total fluid deficit

To find the normal fluid maintenance of 50 ml/kg/24 hrs:

0.9 kg $\times 50$ ml $= 45$ ml total maintenance needs
Total fluid requirement $= $ **153 ml in 24 hrs**

(b) The veterinary surgeon wants the full fluid deficit, plus the fluid maintenance requirements for 6 hrs, to be given over the next 6 hrs. Calculate what this amount will be.
To find the fluid which must be given in 6 hrs:

$$\frac{24 \text{ hrs}}{6 \text{ hrs}} = 4 \text{ (i.e. in } \tfrac{1}{4} \text{ of 24 hrs)}$$

Total maintenance per 24 hrs is 45 ml. Divide this amount by 4:

$$\frac{45 \text{ ml}}{4} = 11.25 \text{ ml total maintenance in 6 hrs}$$

Hedgehog needs 11.25 ml maintenance fluid, plus the total fluid deficit over the next 6 hrs. Therefore add these two totals together:

11.25 ml $+ 108$ ml $= $ **119.25 ml over the next
6 hrs**

Chapter 8

Fluid Therapy – Rates of Administration

These calculations determine the *amount* of fluid administered to a patient over a given *period*. The fluid is controlled by a giving time period set which enables the drip rate to be changed to produce the desired rate. The *flow rate* is usually expressed as *drops/time period* and is known as the *drip rate*.

Calculations normally centre around calculating the drip rate, e.g., 'drops per minute' for a given volume requirement over a period of time. To achieve this calculation the critical data required are:

(1) The volume
(2) The drip factor (a conversion factor indicating how many drops there are in 1 ml)
(3) The relevant time period

With all of these details, the drops/time period can be ascertained.

Examples of typical calculations are illustrated and the preliminary objective on reading the question is to identify the critical details.

Example 1

A 15 kg dog requires 750 ml of an infusion over a 24 hr period. A giving set is used that delivers 20 drops per ml. What drip rate is needed? The answer should give the time (in seconds) for one drop to be delivered.

Answer

Critical details to note:

(1) Fluid required $= 750$ ml
(2) Drip factor of giving set $= 20$ drops per ml
(3) Time period for administration $= 24$ hrs
(4) The body weight is given, but it is not needed for any part of the calculation i.e. it is irrelevant information

The critical detail (1) is the volume requirement of 750 ml. This can be converted into drops using the drip factor.
The critical detail (2) gives a conversion factor for changing ml into drops – i.e. the drip factor, 'the giving set delivers 20 drops per ml'.

750 ml $\times 20$ drops/ml $= 15\,000$ drops

This has to be administered over a 24 hr period – critical detail (3).
From this derived data the number of drops per hr can be calculated

Total number of drops to be administered $= 15\,000$
Total time available to deliver these drops $= 24$ hrs
Therefore drops per hr required to achieve this:

$$= \frac{15\,000}{24} = 625 \text{ drops per hr}$$

drops per minute $= \dfrac{625}{60} = 10.4$ drops/min

Therefore, the giving set is delivering 10.4 drops every 60 seconds. For practical purposes it may be necessary to find the frequency of the drops:

$$= \frac{60 \text{ seconds}}{10.4 \text{ drops}}$$

$= 5.8$ seconds

i.e. **1 drop every 5.8 seconds (s)**

Example 2

A 30 kg dog requires 1500 ml of an infusion over a 24 hr period. The giving set provided has a drip factor of 15 drops /ml. Calculate the flow rate to the patient in drops/minute.

Answer

The first calculation is to convert the volume prescribed from ml into drops. The conversion factor is given in the question as 15 drops for every ml of solution.

Therefore 1500 ml converts to: $1500 \text{ ml} \times \dfrac{15 \text{ drops}}{1 \text{ ml}}$

$= 22\,500$ drops (notice the ml units cancel out)

The patient needs 22 500 drops every 24 hrs

this converts to $\dfrac{22\,500 \text{ drops}}{24 \text{ hrs}} = 937.5$ drops/hr

which in turn converts to $\dfrac{937.5 \text{ drops}}{60 \text{ min}} = 15.6$ drops/min

Note that as this question requires the final answer as drops per minute, the final step of converting how often each drop is delivered is not taken.

Example 3

A dehydrated 20 kg Collie cross-breed is receiving an infusion at the rate of 10 drops per minute for a 24 hr period. The drip factor is 12 drops per ml. Calculate the amount of fluid received by the patient over the day.

Answer

Here, the question has been reversed as usually questions are framed to calculate the drops per minute. This question starts with this data and requires the calculation of the volume. It is designed to ensure that manipulation of the units involved is understood.

Note also that even in such a short question there is still some irrelevant information, i.e. the weight of the patient, although this is given, plays no part in the calculation.

Step 1

Convert the 24 hr period into minutes. This is done to align the time units, minutes (min), with the rate at which the infusion is being delivered, given in the question as 10 drops/min.

$$24\,\text{hrs} = 24 \times 60\,\text{min} = 1440\,\text{min}$$

Now that the drip rate and time period have similar units, they can be multiplied together to give the number of drops administered over 24 hrs.

i.e. $1440\,\text{min} \times \dfrac{10\,\text{drops}}{1\,\text{min}} = 14\,400\,\text{drops}$

(the minutes cancel out – leaving drops as the unit)

Step 2

To convert the number of drops administered over the course of 1 day (24 hrs) to ml, all that is required is the number of drops in 1 ml of infusion.

To convert drops to ml, all that needs to be done is to divide the drops calculated above by the conversion factor of 12 drops per ml (given in the question).

Hence, $\dfrac{14\,400\,\text{drops}}{12\,\text{drops/ml}} = $ **1200 ml will be administered to the patient over 24 hrs**

Example 4

A very dehydrated 20 kg dog is placed on an intravenous drip at 1.5 times the maintenance rate (maintenance = 50 ml/kg/ 24 hrs). What is the total daily volume required, and what would the drip rate be if the giving set delivers 20 drops/ml?

Answer

In this question the *weight of the patient is vital* because it is needed to calculate the volume of fluid required by the patient. In the previous examples the volume was already given, thus making the weight factor irrelevant information.

The question gives this crucial information:
Maintenance $= 50$ ml/kg/24 hrs

This conveys volume information (ml), with the patient's body weight (kg) and connects this information to a time period (hrs). The question also states that 'maintenance' is not sufficient for this patient and that 1.5 times the maintenance rate must be administered.

Step 1

Calculate the volume required by the dog within the 24 hr period.

Given maintenance $= 50$ ml/kg/24 hrs
Body weight $= 20$ kg
Maintenance $= 50$ ml $\times 20$ kg $= 1000$ ml
1.5 maintenance $= 1000$ ml $\times 1.5 = \textbf{1500 ml per day}$

Step 2

Drip factor $= 20$ drops/ml

1500 ml converts to 1500 ml $\times \dfrac{20 \text{ drops}}{\text{ml}} = 30\,000$ drops

These drops have to be given over a 24 hr period
24 hrs $= 24 \times 60$ min $= 1440$ min

Therefore the drip rate i.e. the number of drops/min that need to be given in order to ensure that the patient receives 30 000 drops over 1440 min is calculated by

$$\frac{\text{total number of drops}}{\text{the total time available in min}} = \frac{30\,000}{1440}$$
$$= \textbf{21 drops per min}$$

Example 5

What drip rate would be required for a dehydrated 2 kg Chihuahua bitch that required 150 ml of fluid over a 12 hr period, given a conversion factor of 10 drops/ml for the infusion being used?

Answer

There is no need to calculate the volume as it is given in the question. The weight of the dog is irrelevant as there is no maintenance statement which relies on weight, hence this is irrelevant data.

Convert the volume to drops using the drip factor 10 drops per ml

This gives $150 \, \text{ml} \times \dfrac{10 \, \text{drops}}{\text{ml}} = 1500 \, \text{drops}$

Notice that the period of time allowed to get this infusion into the patient is only 12 hrs.

$12 \, \text{hrs} = 12 \times 60 \, \text{min} = 720 \, \text{min}$

$\text{Drops per minute} = \dfrac{1500 \, \text{drops}}{720 \, \text{min}} = 2.08 \, \text{drops/min}$

$= \mathbf{2 \, drops/min}$ in practical terms

Self-test exercise
(fully-worked answers at the end of this chapter)

(i)   A large dog is brought into the surgery dehydrated, after being left in a car for too long. It has been decided that 3000 ml of infusion must be administered as quickly as possible. Is this achieved faster

(a)   by using a giving set with a 20 drops/ml drip factor and a drip rate of 1 drop every 2 seconds? Or

(b)   by using a giving set with a 15 drops/ml drip factor and a drip rate of 20 drops/min?

(ii)   The given maintenance factor is 50 ml/kg/24 hrs and a 14 kg dog needs 50% maintenance. Calculate what volume, in ℓ, the vet has prescribed for the dog.

(iii)   How long would it take to deliver 2000 ml of fluid to a dog if the giving set delivers 15 drops/ml and the drip rate is 20 drops/min?

(iv)   A 40 kg ewe requires fluid at the rate of 60 ml/kg/24 hrs.
    (a)   By what factor must this original volume be increased if 3600 ml were required for a very dehydrated ewe?
    (b)   If the conversion of ml to drops is 10, what will the giving set have to deliver to administer the 3600 ml in 24 hrs?

(v)   A drip rate of 1 drop every 3 seconds is required to sustain a poodle puppy suffering from excessive heat-stroke. If it is to receive 300 ml of fluid, how long will it take to deliver this if the drip factor is 15 drops per ml?

(vi)   A baby elephant was found distressed and dehydrated, on the plains of the Kruger Valley Safari Park. It required 7 ℓ of fluid in 15 hrs to give it a chance of survival. The drip factor of the giving set is 15 drops/ml.
    (a)   Calculate the drip rate to drops per second required to accomplish this task.
    (b)   What would this drip rate to drops per second reduce to, if the time allowed was 20 hrs and all other factors remained the same?

(vii)   Calculate the frequency of the drops required to deliver the following volumes in 24 hrs using a giving set with a drip factor of 15 drops/ml.
    (a)   960 ml
    (b)   1440 ml
    (c)   1960 ml
    (d)   2400 ml

(viii) At a safari park, a lion cub has been neglected by its mother and the attendant veterinary surgeon has decided that it needs rehydration with dextrose saline before being bottle fed.

This is administered by an intravenous drip at 1.5 times maintenance.

The cub weighs 32 kg and the maintenance rate is 50 ml/kg/24 hrs.

The giving set delivers 15 drops/ml.

Calculate the frequency of the drops.

(ix) In order to administer a solution of 1920 ml over a 24 hr period with a giving set of 20 drops/ml, what would the frequency of the drops need to be?

(x) A dehydrated male ferret weighing 800 g needs an infusion of 90 ml administered over a 2 hr period. The giving set has a drip factor of 10 drops per ml.

    (a) Calculate the flow rate required to achieve this.

    (b) Would this flow rate change if the ferret weighed 700 g? (explain your answer)

    (c) State how the time would be affected if the volume required was 180 ml and the drip rate was increased to 25 drops/min.

Answers to self-test exercises

(i) This is a comparative question and as such can be formatted into two columns to compare the answers.

	Scenario 1	Scenario 2
Volume in ml	3000	3000
Drip factor	20 drops/ml	15 drops/ml
Drops	60 000	45 000
Drops/min	30	20
Min required	2000	2250

Answer: the fluid to use is that described in scenario 1.
1 drop every 2 seconds (s): to calculate the drip rate, divide 60 s (1 min) by 2 s to give the number of drops in 1 min:

$$\frac{60\,s}{2\,s} = 30 \; drops \; per \; min$$

(ii)   Maintenance is 50 ml/kg/24 hrs and the dog weighs 14 kg.

Therefore, volume $= 14\,kg \times 50\,ml = 700\,ml$
50% of 700 ml $= 350\,ml$

The answer is required in ℓ (i.e. 1000 ml)

Therefore $\dfrac{350\,ml}{1000\,ml}$
(i.e. move decimal point 3 places to the left)
Answer: volume $= \mathbf{0.35\,\ell}$

(iii)   2000 ml of fluid delivered to a dog, with a giving set delivering 15 drops/ml.

Therefore 2000 ml $\times$ 15 drops $= 30\,000$ drops

The drip rate is 20 drops per minute, therefore:

$$\frac{30\,000 \; drops}{20 \; drops/min} = 1500\,min$$

There are 60 min per hr, therefore:

$$\frac{1500\,min}{60\,min} = 25\,hrs$$
Answer $= \mathbf{25\,hrs}$ to deliver 2000 ml of fluid

(iv)   A 40 kg ewe needs 60 ml/kg/24 hrs, therefore

$40\,kg \times 60\,ml = 2400\,ml$

(a) If a ewe was very dehydrated and needed 3600 ml:
To find the factor that the original volume must be increased by:

$$\frac{3600\,ml}{2400\,ml} = \mathbf{1.5}$$

2400 ml × 1.5 = 3600 ml
Answer: **the factor is 1.5**

(b) The conversion of ml to drops is 10 (i.e. giving set delivers 10 drops/ml)
The ewe needs 3600 ml over 24 hrs
To find the number of drops:

3600 ml × 10 = 36 000 drops

To find the number of min in 24 hrs:

24 hrs × 60 mins = 1440 min
i.e. 3600 ml need to be delivered in 1440 min

To find how many ml need to be delivered per min:

$$\frac{3600\,ml}{1440\,min} = 2.5\,ml/min$$

Giving set delivers 10 drops per ml
To find the number of drops per min:

2.5 ml × 10 drops = **25 drops/min**

Alternatively, divide the number of drops by the number of minutes:

$$\frac{36\,000\,drops}{1440\,min} = \mathbf{25\ drops/min}$$

Note

To check answer:
drip given over 1440 min × 25 drops = 36 000 drops, which agrees with original amount of drops calculated.

(v)   Poodle puppy needs 300 ml of fluid at a drip rate of 1 drop every 3 s, using a giving set with a drip factor of 15 drops per ml.
To find the number of drops:

$$300 \text{ ml} \times 15 \text{ drops per ml} = 4500 \text{ drops}$$

To find the number of seconds:

$$4500 \text{ drops} \times 3 \text{ seconds} = 13\,500 \text{ s}$$

To find the number of min, divide the total number of s by 60 s (i.e. number of s in 1 min):

$$\frac{13\,500 \text{ s}}{60 \text{ s}} = 225 \text{ min}$$

To find the number of hrs, divide the total number of min by 60 min (i.e. number of min in 1 hr):

$$\frac{225 \text{ min}}{60 \text{ min}} = \mathbf{3.75\,hrs}$$

(vi)   Baby elephant requires 7 ℓ of fluid in 15 hrs. The drip factor of the giving set is 15 drops/ml.

    (a)   To calculate the drip rate:
First turn litres into ml:

$$7 \,\ell \times 1000 \text{ ml} = 7000 \text{ ml}$$

To find the number of drops:

$$7000 \text{ ml} \times 15 \text{ drops/ml} = 105\,000 \text{ drops}$$

To find the number of min, multiply the number of hrs by 60 min (i.e. number of min in 1 hr):

$$15 \text{ hrs} \times 60 \text{ min} = 900 \text{ min}$$

To find the number of s, multiply the number of min by 60 min (i.e. number of s in 1 min):

$$900 \text{ min} \times 60 \text{ s} = 54\,000 \text{ s}$$

To find the number of drops per s, divide the total number of drops needed by the total number of s:

$$\frac{105\,000 \text{ drops}}{54\,000 \text{ s}} = \textbf{1.94 drops/s}$$

i.e. **2 drops/s** for practical purposes

(b) Time is increased to 20 hrs but all other factors are the same, what is the new drip rate?
To find the new drip rate:

$$20 \text{ hrs} = 72\,000 \text{ s}$$
$$\frac{105\,000 \text{ drops}}{72\,000 \text{ s}} = \textbf{1.46 drops/s}$$

i.e. **1.5 drops/s** for practical purposes

(vii) Drip factor remains constant at 15 drops/ml, as does the time at 24 hrs.
The drip rate is to be calculated for each of the following volumes:

(a) 960 ml
To find the number of drops:

960 ml × 15 drops/ml = 14 400 drops

To find the number of min in 24 hrs:

24 hrs × 60 min = 1440 min

To find the number of drops per min:

$$\frac{14\,400 \text{ drops}}{1440 \text{ min}} = 10 \text{ drops per min (i.e. every 60 s)}$$

To find the frequency of the drops:

$$\frac{60 \text{ s}}{10 \text{ drops}} = \textbf{1 drop every 6 s}$$

Calculate answers (b), (c) and (d) in the same way

(b) *Answer* = 15 drops per min = **1 drop every 4 s**

(c) *Answer* = 20.4 drops per min
= **1 drop every 2.9 (i.e. 3) s**

(d)   *Answer* = 25 drops per min
        = **1 drop every 2.4 (i.e. 2.5) s**

(viii)   Lion cub weighing 32 kg needs fluid at 1.5 times the maintenance rate of 50 ml/kg/24 hrs.
   To find the volume of fluid needed over 24 hrs:

   $32\,kg \times 50\,ml = 1600\,ml$ over 24 hrs

   Needs 1.5 × the maintenance rate:

   $1600\,ml \times 1.5 = 2400\,ml$

   To find the number of drops:

   $2400\,ml \times 15\,drops = 36\,000\,drops$

   To find the number of minutes:

   $24\,hrs \times 60\,min = 1440\,min$

   To find the number of drops per min:

   $$\frac{36\,000\,drops}{1440\,min} = 25\,drops/min$$

   To find the frequency of the drops

   $$\frac{60\,s}{25\,drops} = 2.4\,s$$
   = **1 drop every 2.4 s**

(ix)   Administer 1920 ml over 24 hrs with a giving set of 20 drops/ml. What is the drip rate.
   To find the number of drops:

   $1920\,ml \times 20\,drops = 38\,400\,drops$ over 24 hrs

   To find the number of minutes the fluid is given over:

   $24\,hrs \times 60\,min = 1440\,min$

To find the number of drops per min:

$$\frac{38\,400 \text{ drops}}{1440 \text{ min}} = 26.66 \text{ drops/min}$$

(i.e. 27 drops in practical terms)

To find the frequency of the drops:

$$\frac{60 \text{ s}}{27 \text{ drops}} = \mathbf{2.2\,s}$$

i.e. **1 drop every 2.2 seconds**

(x)   800 g ferret needs 90 ml of fluid over 2 hrs, using a giving set with a drip factor of 10 drops per ml.

(a)   To find the number of drops:

$$90 \text{ ml} \times 10 \text{ drops} = 900 \text{ drops}$$

To find the number of minutes:

$$2 \text{ hrs} \times 60 \text{ min} = 120 \text{ min}$$

To find the number of drops per minute:

$$\frac{900 \text{ drops}}{120 \text{ min}} = 7.5 \text{ drops per minute (8 drops per minute in practical terms)}$$

To find the frequency of the drops:

$$\frac{60 \text{ s}}{8 \text{ drops}} = 1 \text{ drop every } 7.5 \text{ s (i.e. } \mathbf{8\,s} \text{ in practical terms)}$$

(b)   Answer no, as the weight has not featured as a key factor in the flow rate calculation.

(c)   Fluid volume has doubled to 180 ml, given at 25 drops per min.
Giving set still at 10 drops per ml

To find the number of drops:

$$180 \text{ ml} \times 10 \text{ drops per ml} = 1800 \text{ drops}$$

To find the number of minutes that the infusion is given over:

$$\frac{1800 \text{ drops}}{25 \text{ drops/min}} = 72 \text{ minutes}$$

Answer: 72 minutes, i.e. it would take **48 minutes less** to deliver twice the amount at 25 drops per min.

Chapter 9

Anaesthetic Gases – Flow Rates

This section focuses on the calculations involved in determining the flow rates required to administer anaesthetic gases to patients. There are several sub-calculations involved in this process which need to be learnt and mastered, in order to calculate the gas flow rates. These calculations involve:

(1)   Tidal volume
(2)   Respiratory rate
(3)   Minute volume
(4)   Circuit factor

Tidal volume

The volume of gas inhaled or exhaled during each respiratory cycle multiplied by the body weight. It is expressed in ml/kg and for a cat or dog is usually in the range of 10–15 ml/kg.

Respiratory rate

The number of inspirations taken each minute. In the dog, this is about 10–30 respirations/min and in the cat, about 20–30. Normally a heavier animal would inhale/exhale more slowly than a lighter animal.

Minute volume

The tidal volume multiplied by the respiratory rate per min, i.e. the total amount of air inhaled/exhaled in 1 min.

Circuit factor

The factor to be applied to the calculation is dependent upon the type of anaesthetic circuit in use. The weight of the patient is a determining factor in the type of circuit. Where there is a range given for a circuit factor, e.g. 2.0–3.0, (see table 9.1) and there is a choice of circuit factor, ideally the middle of the range or the highest factor should be chosen. In an examination question, the circuit factor may be given, or optional. Therefore, the circuit factors should be learnt as they may need to be inserted into a calculation. Another consideration of circuit choice is the size of the patient's lungs. A slim, deep-chested dog such as a greyhound may weigh less, but have a larger lung capacity than, for example, an overweight Labrador retriever.

Table 9.1 Anaesthetic circuit table

Circuit type	Circuit factor	Weight of patient in kg
Ayres T-Piece	2.0–3.0	up to 8
Bain	2.0–3.0	8–30
Circle	1.0	20 kg or more
Lack or Magill	1.0–1.5	8–60
To & Fro	1.0	15 kg or more

Flow rate is calculated by multiplying the minute volume by the circuit factor:

flow rate = minute volume × circuit factor

NB: The unit of flow rate in relation to the body weight of the patient is ml/kg/min

Example 1

Calculate the flow rate required for an 8 kg dog using an Ayres T-piece. Assume a respiratory rate of 20 respirations/min.

Answer

First calculate tidal volume (as the minute volume depends on this):

tidal volume = body weight × volume of gas inhaled/exhaled
per kg during each respiratory cycle (in this
case use 15 ml/kg)
= 8 kg × 15 ml/kg = 120 ml

Then calculate minute volume:

minute volume = tidal volume × respiratory rate
(given as 20 respirations/min)
Therefore, minute volume = 120 ml × 20
= 2400 ml/min

Then calculate flow rate:

flow rate = minute volume × circuit factor
= 2400 ml/min × 2.5
= 6000 ml/min

NB: 2.5 circuit factor is chosen as Ayres T-piece is to be used for an 8 kg patient and 2.5 is the mid point in the range 2.0–3.0.

Divide the flow rate by the patient's body weight in kg to express the flow rate in ml/kg/min

The flow rate would then be expressed as

$$\frac{6000\,\text{ml/min}}{8\,\text{kg}} = \textbf{750 ml/kg/min}$$

Example 2

Calculate the flow rate required for a 25 kg dog using a Magill circuit. Assume a respiratory rate of 15 respirations/min.

Answer

(1) Calculate the tidal volume
(2) Calculate the minute volume
(3) Calculate the flow rate

(1) Tidal volume $= 10$ ml/kg $\times$ body weight
            $= 10$ ml/kg $\times 25$ kg $= 250$ ml
    (10 ml/kg was selected as, at 25 kg, this is a reasonably large dog)

(2) Minute volume $=$ tidal volume $\times$ respiratory rate
                $= 250$ ml $\times 15$ respirations/min
                $= 3750$ ml/min

    Circuit factor $= 1.5$ (as Magill's factor not given so higher end of range chosen)

(3) Flow rate $=$ minute volume $\times$ circuit factor
            $= 3750$ ml/min $\times 1.5$
            $= 5625$ ml/min

To express this flow rate in relation to the body weight of the patient, divide the flow rate by the body weight to determine the flow rate in ml/kg/min.

$$\frac{5625\,\text{ml/min}}{25\,\text{kg}} = \textbf{225 ml/kg/min}$$

Example 3

Calculate the flow rate mix required of oxygen and nitrous oxide for a 25 kg dog, to be maintained on a Magill circuit (assume a tidal volume of 250 ml) and use a circuit factor of 1.35.

Oxygen is 33% of the mix. Respiratory rate is 20 respirations/min.

Select from:

(a)   1.25 ℓ oxygen : 2.50 ℓ nitrous oxide
(b)   1.75 ℓ oxygen : 3.25 ℓ nitrous oxide
(c)   2.25 ℓ oxygen : 4.50 ℓ nitrous oxide
(d)   2.75 ℓ oxygen : 5.50 ℓ nitrous oxide

Answer

It may be thought that the 33% mix of oxygen is a clue to the answer and that by calculating the % composition of each mix first, it gives a quick route to the answer. If there were only one answer which gave a 33% split to the oxygen in the mixture then the correct selection would be obvious. However, all the ratios of the gases give a similar answer.

The quickest way to the answer is to calculate it:

Tidal volume = 250 ml, given in question
(check: 25 kg weight × 10 ml as recommended = 250 ml)
Respiratory rate = 20 respirations/min
Circuit factor = 1.35, given

Minute volume = tidal volume × respiratory rate
= 250 ml × 20 respirations/min
= 5000 ml/min

Flow rate = minute volume × circuit factor
= 5000 ml/min × 1.35
= 6750 ml/min

Therefore, if the flow rate is 6750 ml/min and the required mix contains 33% oxygen, then the oxygen content can be calculated by dividing by 100 to get the representative figure for 1% then multiplying by 33 to obtain a figure for 33%.

$$\text{The oxygen content is } \frac{33}{100} \times 6750 \,\text{ml} = 2227.5 \,\text{ml of oxygen}$$

i.e. for every 100 ml of gaseous mixture, 33 ml is oxygen and 67 ml is nitrous oxide.

In 6750 ml of mixture there are 2227.5 ml of oxygen.

Therefore the mix is **2.23 ℓ of oxygen : 4.52 ℓ of nitrous oxide**

The nearest answer to this mixture is answer **(c)**.

Example 4

What flow rate is required for a male Weimaraner weighing 66lb: it is geriatric and has a respiratory rate of 20 respirations/min?

A Circle circuit is in use with a circuit factor of 1.0.

What would the rate be if the dog were a Newfoundland weighing 154 lb, and all other factors remained constant?

Answer

The patient's weight is expressed in lb (pounds), which must first be converted to kg.

The question is comparative and lends itself to a tabular form of answer as follows:

First establish the weight of the patient in kg using 1 kg = 2.2 lb

$$\text{Weight of first dog} = \frac{66}{2.2}\,\text{kg} = 30\,\text{kg}$$
$$\text{Weight of second dog} = \frac{154}{2.2}\,\text{kg} = 70\,\text{kg}$$

Next create a simple table:

Weight kg	30	70	
Tidal volume ml/kg resp. cycle	10	10	(see beginning of chapter)
Respiratory rate	20	20	(respirations/min (given))
Circuit factor	1.0	1.0	(given)
Tidal volume total ml	300	700	(body weight × tidal volume ml/kg)
Minute volume ml/min	6000	14 000	(tidal volume × respiratory rate)
Flow rate ml/min	6000	14 000	(minute volume × circuit factor)
Flow rate ml/kg/min	200	200	(flow rate ml/min divided by body weight)

Example 5

A 20 kg dog is to be anaesthetised; its minute volume is known to be 4.5 ℓ/min. A Lack circuit is being used with a circuit factor of 1.5. Which one of the following is the flow rate?

(a) 6075 ml/min
(b) 6570 ml/min
(c) 6750 ml/min
(d) 7650 ml/min

Answer

The weight is irrelevant when answering this question. A simple multiplication of the minute volume × circuit factor (both given in the question) provides the flow rate.

Hence 4.5 ℓ/min × 1.5 circuit factor = 6.75 ℓ/min converted to ml by multiplying by 1000 (Note: 1000 ml = 1 ℓ)

= 6.75 ℓ/min × 1000 = **6750 ml/min**

NB: If the flow rate then needs to be expressed in relation to the body weight, divide the flow rate by 20 kg which is given in the question.

$$\text{Therefore } \frac{6750\,\text{ml/min}}{20\,\text{kg}} = 337.5\,\text{ml/kg/min}$$

Self-test exercise
(fully-worked answers at the end of this chapter)

(i)   A 4 kg cat needs to be anaesthetised. Its tidal volume lies within the normal range.

Calculate the minute volume and flow rate required using an Ayres T-piece and a circuit factor of 3.

Respiratory rate is 25 respirations/min.

Also express the flow rate in ml/kg/min.

(ii)   Calculate the flow rates for the two dogs whose details are listed below:

Name	Mutton	Jeff
Weight	132 lb	3 kg
Tidal volume	10 ml/kg	15 ml/kg
Respiratory rate	10	20 respirations/min
Circuit factor	1.25	3.00

Compare the flow rates per kg/min for the two dogs.

(iii)   A hedgehog has been injured in an RTA and needs to be anaesthetised.

What data would you require in order to calculate the flow rate?

The hedgehog weighs 1.5 kg. From the information at the beginning of the chapter, work out the rest of the data required and calculate the flow rate both in ℓ/min and as ml/kg/min.

(iv)   Calculate the circuit factor required to obtain a flow rate of 20.25 ℓ per min using a Bain circuit when anaesthetising a 30 kg dog. The respiratory rate is 15 respirations/min.

(v) Calculate the flow rate in ml/min required for a 55 kg Great Dane using a Magill circuit. The respiratory rate is 10 respirations/min.

(vi) Calculate the flow rate mix required of oxygen and nitrous oxide for a 50 kg dog, to be maintained on a Magill circuit (assume a tidal volume of 500 ml) and use a circuit factor of 1.35.

Oxygen is 33% of the mix and the respiratory rate is 10 respirations/min.

Which one of the following is the correct flow rate mix?

(a) 1.50 ℓ oxygen : 3.05 ℓ nitrous oxide
(b) 2.25 ℓ oxygen : 6.78 ℓ nitrous oxide
(c) 2.23 ℓ oxygen : 4.52 ℓ nitrous oxide
(d) 2.75 ℓ oxygen : 5.50 ℓ nitrous oxide

(vii) What flow rate is required for a 33 lb dog with a respiratory rate of 15 respirations/min. A Lack circuit is in use with a circuit factor of 1.5.

What would the rate be if the dog weighed 99 lb and all other factors remained constant ?

(viii) Express the following flow rates in ℓ/min

450 ml/kg/min for a 2 kg patient
300 ml/kg/min for a 15 kg patient
200 ml/kg/min for a 30 kg patient
100 ml/kg/min for a 60 kg patient

(ix) Express the following litre flow rates as ml/kg/min

5.0 ℓ/min for a 16 kg patient
7.5 ℓ/min for a 30 kg patient
9.0 ℓ/min for a 90 kg patient
1.5 ℓ/min for a 4 kg patient

(x) A 40 kg dog needs to be anaesthetised. Its tidal volume lies within the normal 10–15 ml/kg range.

Calculate the minute volume and flow rate in ml/min required using a Magill circuit with a circuit factor of 1.5.

Respiratory rate is 10 respirations/min.
Also express the flow rate in ml/kg/min.

Answers to self-test exercise

(i)   Body weight $= 4$ kg
      Tidal volume $= 4$ kg $\times 15$ ml/kg (see beginning of chapter)
              $= 60$ ml
      Minute volume $=$ tidal volume $\times$ respiratory rate
              $= 60$ ml $\times 25$ respirations/min
              $= 1500$ ml/min
      Flow rate $=$ circuit factor $\times$ minute volume
              $= 3 \times 1500$ ml $= 4500$ ml/min

      Can also be expressed as $\dfrac{4500 \text{ ml}}{4 \text{ kg}} = \mathbf{1125\ ml/kg/min}$

(ii) This question was given as a table and it can also be
      answered in tabular form:

Name	Mutton	Jeff
Weight kg	60	3
Tidal volume in ml/kg	10	15
Tidal volume total ml	600	45
Respiratory rate breaths/minute	10	20
Minute volume ml/min	6000	900
Circuit factor	1.25	3.00
Flow rate ml/min	**7500**	**2700**
Flow rate ml/kg/min	**125**	**900**

(iii) Only one piece of data is given and the rest is standard
      information.
      Calculate the tidal volume, which is body weight $\times$ volume
      of gas inhaled/exhaled per kg during each respiratory
      cycle.
      This is 1.5 kg $\times 15$ ml/kg (choose 15 ml as small animal)
      Tidal volume $= 22.5$ ml

Respiratory rate = 30 respirations/min (assumed as smaller animal breathes faster than a larger one)

Minute volume = tidal volume × respiratory rate

= 22.5 ml × 30 respirations/min

= 675 ml/min

Flow rate = minute volume × circuit factor

= 675 ml/min × 3 (highest factor in the range for an Ayres T-piece)

= 2025 ml/min

Expressed as ml/kg/min

$$\frac{2025\,\text{ml/min}}{1.5\,\text{kg}} = \textbf{1350 ml/kg/min}$$

(iv) This question is unusual as it requires the circuit factor to be calculated.

(This type of question is likely to arise in an examination in order to check understanding of the mechanics of the formulas – however, as the circuit factors should be learnt, it should be easy to recognise a reasonable answer.)

Flow rate = 20.25 ℓ/min = 20 250 ml/min

(NB: 20.25 ℓ × 1000 = 20 250 ml)

Tidal volume = 30 kg × 15 ml/kg (volume of gas inhaled/exhaled per kg per respiratory cycle)

= 450 ml

Minute volume = tidal volume × respirations/min

= 450 ml × 15 respirations/min

= 6750 ml/min

Flow rate = minute volume × circuit factor

Therefore circuit factor = $\dfrac{\text{flow rate}}{\text{minute volume}}$

= $\dfrac{20\,250\,\text{ml/min}}{6750\,\text{ml/min}}$

Answer = **3** (a reasonable answer as a Bain circuit has a factor in the range of 2.0–3.0)

(v)   Body weight = 55 kg
        Tidal volume = 55 kg × 10 ml/kg (assumed)
                    = 550 ml
        Respiratory rate = 10 respirations/min
        Minute volume = tidal volume × respiratory rate
                    = 550 ml × 10 respirations/min
                    = 5500 ml/min
        Circuit factor (Magill) assume 1.5
        Flow rate = minute volume × circuit factor
                    = 5500 ml/min × 1.5
                    = **8250 ml/min**

(vi)   Tidal volume = 500 ml, given in question
        (check: 50 kg weight × 10 ml/kg as recommended
        = 500 ml)
        Respiratory rate = 10 respirations/min
        Circuit factor = 1.35, given
        Minute volume = tidal volume × respiratory rate
                    = 500 ml × 10 respirations/min
                    = 5000 ml/min
        Flow rate = minute volume × circuit factor
                    = 5000 ml/min × 1.35
                    = 6750 ml/min

Therefore if the flow rate is 6750 ml/min and the required mix contains 33% oxygen, the oxygen content can be calculated by dividing by 100 to get the representative figure for 1%, then multiplying by 33 to get a figure for 33%.

The oxygen content is $\dfrac{33}{100} \times 6750\,\text{ml} = 2227.5\,\text{ml of oxygen}$

i.e. for every 100 ml of gaseous mixture, 33 ml is oxygen and 67 ml is nitrous oxide.

In 6750 ml of mixture there are 2227.5 ml of oxygen. Therefore the mix is **2.23 ℓ of oxygen : 4.52 ℓ of nitrous oxide**

Answer = **(c)**

(vii)   To answer this question, first change the weight from lb to kg as the units must be the same in order to compare the data and the answers.

$$\text{Therefore } 33\,\text{lb} = \frac{33\,\text{lb}}{2.2} = 15\,\text{kg and}$$
$$99\,\text{lb} = \frac{99\,\text{lb}}{2.2} = 45\,\text{kg}$$

Then create a simple comparison chart

Weight kg	15	45
Tidal volume ml/kg	15	10
Tidal volume total ml	225	450
Respirations/min	15	15 (given)
Minute volume ml	3375	6750
Circuit factor	1.5	1.5
Flow rate ml/min	**5062.5**	**10 125**
Flow rate ml/kg/min	**337.5**	**225**

(viii)

Flow rate ml/kg/min	Weight kg (given)	Answer ℓ/min
450	2	$\dfrac{450 \times 2}{1000} = 0.9$
300	15	$\dfrac{300 \times 15}{1000} = 4.5$
200	30	$\dfrac{200 \times 30}{1000} = 6.0$
100	60	$\dfrac{100 \times 60}{1000} = 6.0$

(ix)

Flow rate ℓ/min (given)	Weight kg (given)	ml/kg/min
5.0	16	$\dfrac{5.0 \times 1000}{16} = 312.5$
7.5	30	$\dfrac{7.5 \times 1000}{30} = 250.0$

| 9.0 | 90 | $\dfrac{9.0 \times 1000}{90} = 100.0$ |
| 1.5 | 4 | $\dfrac{1.5 \times 1000}{4} = 375.0$ |

(x)   A 40 kg dog needs anaesthetising. As the minute volume relies on the tidal volume, calculate this first,

i.e. tidal volume = body weight × 10–15 ml/kg

(as this is a large dog use 10 ml/kg)

Tidal volume = 40 kg × 10 ml/kg = 400 ml

Minute volume = tidal volume × respiratory rate

(given at 10 respirations/min)

Therefore minute volume = 400 ml × 10

= **4000 ml/min**

Flow rate = minute volume × circuit factor

(circuit factor is given as 1.5 for the Magill)

= 4000 ml/min × 1.5

= **6000 ml/min**

To express this as ml/kg/min, take

$$\frac{\text{flow rate}}{\text{body weight}} = \frac{6000\,\text{ml/min}}{40\,\text{kg}} = \textbf{150ml/kg/min}$$

Chapter 10

Radiography

This chapter explains how to carry out the basic calculations which are necessary in order to ensure that the maximum benefit is obtained from the use of X-ray machines.

Terminology

The use of prefixes such as kilo- and milli- are explained fully in Chapter 1 but where appropriate a brief explanation has been included in this section.

Kilovoltage (kV)

Kilovoltage refers to how many thousands of volts are applied across the X-ray tube, e.g. 100 kV means 100 thousand volts are applied.

Note

kV is written with a small k (kilo) and a large V (volt). Changing the kV is the most effective method of changing the contrast. The higher the kV, the greater the penetrating power of the X-ray beam will be.

Milliamperage (mA)

Milliamperage refers to the current flowing through the X-ray tube.

The flow of electricity is measured in amperes (A) (often abbreviated to amps)

The mA setting determines the intensity of the X-ray beam.

200 mA means the current flowing is 200 thousandths of an ampere.

Note

mA is written with a small m and a large A.

Milliampere–seconds (mAs)

The exposure time is measured in seconds (s). Thus the product of the current flowing and the exposure time will reflect the amount of X-rays produced. Changing the mAs affects the density of the radiograph.

Note

mAs is written with a small m (milli), a large A (ampere) and a small s (second).

Examples of mAs

200 mA × 1 s = 200 mAs
800 mA × 0.25 s = 200 mAs
20 mA × 1 s = 20 mAs
20 mA × 0.5 s = 10 mAs

The aim is to use an exposure time (s) which is as low as possible (among other beneficial effects, this will reduce the risk of blurring due to movement). From the above examples it can be seen that in order to keep the mAs constant, reducing the exposure time necessitates increasing the mA.

Occasionally in examination questions, time is expressed as fractions of a second rather than as a decimal. In such cases it is best to convert the fraction into its decimal equivalent (by dividing the top of the fraction by the bottom) before calculating the mAs.

Example 1

Calculate the mAs produced by the following settings:

(i)   100 mA and $\frac{1}{2}$ s

(ii)   250 mA and $\frac{1}{20}$ s

(iii)   300 mA and $\frac{1}{5}$ s

Answer

(i)   100 mA $\times$ 0.5 s = **50 mAs**

(ii)   250 mA $\times$ 0.05 s = **12.5 mAs**

(iii)   300 mA $\times$ 0.2 s = **60 mAs**

Manipulating the formula (see also Chapter 2, Basic Principles)

The standard formula (or equation) is mAs = mA $\times$ s
This allows the mAs to be calculated when the mA and exposure time (s) are known. However, sometimes the mAs and either the exposure time or the mA are known, and the other value has to be calculated. To do this necessitates transposing or manipulating the formula. This process is explained fully in Chapter 2 but, in brief, it involves changing the formula to make mA or s the subject as follows:

$$mAs = mA \times s$$
$$mA = \frac{mAs}{s}$$
$$s = \frac{mAs}{mA}$$

It may be easier to remember the manipulation if it is thought of as a triangle:

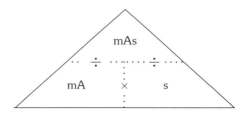

To apply the triangle:

- First put the known information into the appropriate places in the triangle.
- Next cover the part of the triangle which contains the information which has to be found.
- Finally divide or multiply (as appropriate) the remaining visible figures.

Example 2

Calculate the mAs for settings of 50 mA and 0.5 s.

Answer

Place the known information in the triangle and cover the section marked mAs:

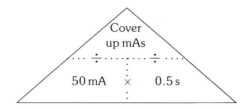

From the triangle, mAs = mA × s

$$= 50\,mA \times 0.5\,s$$
$$= \mathbf{25\,mAs}$$

Example 3

Calculate the exposure time needed to produce 80 mAs when the mA setting is 160.

Answer

Place the known information in the triangle and cover the section marked mAs:

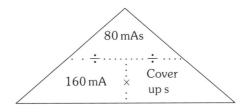

From the triangle, $s = \dfrac{mAs}{mA}$

$$= \dfrac{80\,mAs}{160\,mA}$$
$$= \mathbf{0.5\,s}$$

Example 4

Calculate the mA needed to produce 120 mAs when the exposure time is 0.25 s.

Answer

Place the known information in the triangle and cover the section marked mA:

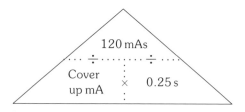

From the triangle, $mA = \dfrac{mAs}{s}$

$$= \dfrac{120\,mAs}{0.25\,s}$$

$$= 480\,mA$$

Combined effects of kV and mAs

The kV and the mAs are linked by a simple rule:

Increasing the kV by 10 allows the mAs to be halved
Decreasing the kV by 10 necessitates doubling the mAs

Example 5

A radiograph is taken using settings of 50 kV and 24 mAs. The next exposure is taken using 60 kV. What should the new mAs setting be if the radiographic density is to be kept the same?

Answer

Increasing the kV by 10 means the mAs must be halved

Therefore the new mAs setting $= \dfrac{24}{2}$

$$= 12\,mAs$$

Example 6

A radiograph is taken using settings of 60 kV and 24 mAs. The next exposure is taken with a setting of 36 mAs. How many kV are required in order to keep the radiographic density the same?

Answer

The mAs has increased by 50% $\left(\dfrac{36-24}{24} \times 100 \right)$

Therefore the kV can be reduced by 5
Therefore **55 kV are required**.

The grid factor

The grid factor is the amount by which the exposure (mAs) must be increased when using a particular grid.

New exposure = old exposure × grid factor

Example 7

The mAs setting for a particular radiograph is 150.
Calculate the new mAs setting if a grid with a factor of 2 is used but all other variables are unchanged.

Answer

New mAs = old mAs × grid factor
= 150 mAs × 2
= **300 mAs**

Film Focal Distance (FFD)

The focal distance between the X-ray head and the film is known as the Film Focal Distance (FFD). Changing the FFD has a dramatic effect upon the intensity of the X-ray beam. The rule is:

The intensity is inversely proportional to the square of the FFD

This is known as the *inverse square law* which, put simply, means that if the FFD is doubled, then the intensity will be reduced to a quarter of its previous value (double the distance = quarter the effect).

The practical implication of this is that if the FFD is changed, the mAs must also be changed to compensate if the radiographic density is to remain the same. To calculate what the new exposure should be, the following formula must be used:

$$\text{new exposure} = \text{old exposure} \times \frac{\text{new FFD}^2}{\text{old FFD}^2}$$

Note

FFD^2 means that FFD is multiplied by itself once
e.g. $4^2 = 4 \times 4 = 16$

Example 8

The exposure settings for a particular radiograph are
FFD = 1200 mm, mAs = 64
The next radiograph is to be taken after the FFD is decreased to 600 mm.
Calculate what the new mAs setting should be if the radiographic density is to remain the same.

Answer

$$\text{New exposure} = \text{old exposure} \times \frac{\text{new FFD}^2}{\text{old FFD}^2}$$

$$= 64 \, \text{mAs} \times \frac{600^2}{1200^2}$$

$$= 64 \, \text{mAs} \times \frac{600 \times 600}{1200 \times 1200}$$

(note the top and bottom can be divided by 600 twice)

$$= 64 \, \text{mAs} \times \tfrac{1}{2} \times \tfrac{1}{2}$$

$$= 64 \, \text{mAs} \times \tfrac{1}{4}$$

$$= \mathbf{16 \, mAs}$$

Note

In this example the figures are simple which means that the calculation could have been carried out by applying the logic that because the FFD has been halved, the intensity will have increased by a factor of 4. Therefore the mAs will have to be reduced to a $\frac{1}{4}$ of its previous value in order to compensate.

Example 9

The exposure settings for a particular radiograph are
FFD $= 700$ mm
mAs $= 64$
The next radiograph is to be taken after the FFD is increased to 1400 mm.
Calculate what the new mAs setting should be if the radiographic density is to remain the same:

Answer

$$\text{New exposure} = \text{old exposure} \times \frac{\text{new FFD}^2}{\text{old FFD}^2}$$
$$= 64 \text{ mAs} \times \frac{1400^2}{700^2}$$
$$= 64 \text{ mAs} \times \frac{1400 \times 1400}{700 \times 700}$$

(note the top and bottom can be divided by 700 twice)

$$= 64 \text{ mAs} \times \frac{2}{1} \times \frac{2}{1}$$
$$= 64 \text{ mAs} \times \frac{4}{1}$$
$$= \mathbf{256\,mAs}$$

Self-test exercise
(fully-worked answers at the end of this chapter)

(i) An exposure requires 30mA, and 2.5 s
Calculate the mAs.

(ii)   Settings of 80 kV, 40 mAs and 16 mA are to be used for a particular radiograph. Calculate the exposure time.

(iii)   The standard exposure (as recorded in the practice expo-sure book) for a radiograph is 60 kV, 15 mA and 0.2 s.
If the original kV setting is increased to 70 kV, what mAs should be used to keep the density of the radiograph constant?

(iv)   After taking a radiograph using 10 mAs and 60 kV you decide to double the radiographic density for a second film. Which exposure should be used?

(a)   200 mA, 0.10 s, 60 kV
(b)   150 mA, 0.20 s, 60 kV
(c)   100 mA, 0.20 s, 70 kV
(d)   300 mA, 0.03 s, 60 kV

(v)   By how much must the mAs be decreased from 40 mAs to halve the radiographic density?

(a)   5 mAs
(b)   10 mAs
(c)   15 mAs
(d)   20 mAs

(vi)   Settings of 80 kV, 40 mAs and 16 mA have been used for a particular radiograph. The kV setting is to be lowered from 80 kV to 60 kV.
Calculate what the new mAs setting should be in order to keep the radiographic density constant.

(vii)   The standard exposure (as stated in the practice exposure book) for a radiograph is 60 kV, 15 mA and 0.2 s at a FFD of 700 mm.
What is the new time setting required in order to maintain the same radiographic density if a grid (with a grid factor of 3.0) is used and the other settings remain the same?

(viii) The standard exposure (as stated in the practice exposure book) for a radiograph is 60 kV, 15 mA and 0.2 s at a FFD of 700 mm.

What is the new time setting required in order to maintain the radiographic density, if a grid (with a grid factor of 2.0) is used and the kV is raised to 70?

(ix) If the FFD is increased from 800 mm to 1600 mm, how must the mAs be adjusted to maintain the same radiographic density?

(a) decreased by a factor of 4
(b) decreased by a factor of 2
(c) increased by a factor of 4
(d) increased by a factor of 2

(x) The exposure settings for a particular radiograph are
FFD = 700mm
mA = 64
exposure time = 1 s
The next radiograph is to be taken with the same mA setting but the FFD halved to 350 mm.
Calculate what the new exposure time should be if radiographic density is to remain the same.

Answers to self-test exercise

(i) $mAs = mA \times s$
$$= 30 \times 2.5$$
$$= \textbf{75 mAs}$$

(ii) $mAs = 40$, $mA = 16$
Therefore $s = \dfrac{mAs}{mA}$
$$= \frac{40}{16}$$
$$= \textbf{2.5 s}$$

(iii)   Original mAs $= 15 \times 0.2 = 3$ mAs
Increasing the kV by 10 requires half the mAs

Therefore new mAs $= \dfrac{3}{2} = \mathbf{1.5\,mAs}$

(iv)   (a)   **60 kV; 200 mA $\times$ 0.10 s $=$ 20 mAs**
              (double the original mAs doubles the radio-
              graphic density)
        (b)   60 kV; 150 mA $\times$ 0.20 s $= 30$ mAs
        (c)   70 kV; 100 mA $\times$ 0.20 s $= 20$ mAs
        (d)   60 kV; 300 mA $\times$ 0.03 s $= 9$ mAs

(v)   Answer (d) because half of 40 mAs $= 20$ mAs

(vi)   Lowering the kV by 20 will reduce the radiographic density by a factor of 4.
Therefore the mAs must be increased by a factor of 4.
Therefore the mAs must be increased from 40 to **160**

(vii)   Original mAs $= 15$ mA $\times$ 0.2 s
                    $= 3$ mAs
New mAs $=$ original mAs $\times$ grid factor
                    $= 3$ mAs $\times$ 3.0 $= 9$ mAs
New time $= \dfrac{9\,\text{mAs}}{15\,\text{mA}}$
                    $= \mathbf{0.6\ s}$

Note

Another way of looking at this problem would be to say that if the mAs increase by a factor of 3 but the mA does not change then the time must increase by a factor of 3

(viii) No change in exposure time will be required because raising the kV by 10 allows the mAs to be halved, but this is offset by the addition of the grid which would necessitate doubling the mAs.

(ix)   The FFD has been doubled, therefore the intensity of the X-ray beam will have been reduced to a $\frac{1}{4}$ of its previous value.

Therefore the mAs will have to be increased by a factor of 4 in order to keep the radiographic density the same.

Therefore, answer = (c)

(x) Original mAs = 64 mA × 1 s

$$= 64 \text{ mAs}$$

The FFD has been halved.

Therefore the intensity of the X-ray beam will have increased by a factor of 4.

Therefore the mAs must be reduced to a $\frac{1}{4}$ of its previous value in order to keep the radiographic density the same.

Therefore the new mAs will be $\dfrac{64}{4}$ mAs = 16 mAs

mAs = mA × s

Therefore new time $= \dfrac{\text{mAs}}{\text{mA}}$

$$= \dfrac{16 \text{ mAs}}{64 \text{ mA}}$$

$$= \dfrac{1}{4} \text{s}$$

$$= \mathbf{0.25\,s}$$

Chapter 11

Value Added Tax (VAT)

Although this book is primarily concerned with the explanation of veterinary calculations, it is likely that veterinary staff will also have to be involved in the administration of VAT. This may be at the reception desk or in dealing with suppliers or clients.

This chapter explains the principles of VAT and describes various methods of calculating it.

VAT is a tax on *turnover*, not on profit and the basic principle is that the VAT should be borne by the *final* consumer. Businesses registered for VAT may deduct the VAT they pay to suppliers from the VAT they collect from clients. The difference must be either paid to, or claimed from, HM Customs and Excise.

There are two common calculations relating to VAT. The first case is where the VAT needs to be calculated on a given amount. The second is where the total amount is known *including* the VAT and there is a need to ascertain the VAT element and the basic amount separately.

The principle of VAT

The illustration below demonstrates the mechanics of collection and handling of VAT. It also shows how:

- VAT is handled at each stage of the transaction
- Customs and Excise gets net VAT from each stage
- the final consumer pays the entire VAT amount

Illustration of how VAT is calculated and charged

This illustration tracks the VAT collected at each transaction during the manufacture and retailing of a desk. It also shows how the VAT is calculated at each stage resulting in the final amount of VAT paid to Customs and Excise.

An estate has surplus wood, which it sells to the local furniture maker for £100 plus VAT.

The furniture maker uses the wood to make a desk and sells it to a local retail shop for £150 plus VAT.

The shop then sells the desk to the final consumer for £300 plus VAT.

The VAT for each of the transactions will be calculated below. The current rate of VAT is 17.5%.

Furniture maker

Pays £100 + 17.5% VAT to the estate for the wood.

As shown in the chapter on percentages (Chapter 2), a percentage means the amount per cent or per hundred.

In other words, for every £100 of goods the supplier buys, he must pay a tax of 17.5% of its value to Customs and Excise. This % can be turned into a money value by dividing the original amount of £100 by 100 to find the value of 1%, then multiplying this answer by 17.5 to calculate the value of 17.5%.

$$\frac{£100}{100} = £1.00 \text{ and } £1.00 \times 17.5 = £17.50$$

Therefore, the furniture maker pays £100 + £17.50 = £117.50 for the wood.

The furniture maker sells the desk to the retailer for £150.00 + VAT = £176.25 (see following calculation).

Furniture retailer

Pays the furniture maker £150 + 17.5% VAT for the desk.

From the illustration above, to calculate the amount of VAT, take the original cost of £150 and divide it by 100. This will establish what 1% of £150 is; multiply by the tax figure 17.5 to calculate what 17.5% of this figure is.

Take $\dfrac{£150}{100} = £1.50 = 1\%$, multiply this by 17.5 to find what 17.5% is

Therefore £1.50 × 17.5 = £26.25 VAT

The total figure the retailer pays the furniture maker is £150 for the desk plus £26.25 VAT

= £176.25

The final customer

Pays the retailer £300 + 17.5% VAT for the desk.

As before, to calculate the VAT, divide the original cost by 100 to establish what 1% is equivalent to

i.e. $\dfrac{£300}{100} = £3.00 = 1\%$

Then multiply by 17.5 to calculate the VAT, i.e. £3.00 × 17.5 = £52.50 VAT.

Therefore, the total paid by the customer is £300 for the desk plus £52.50 VAT = £352.50

This is what the final consumer pays: **£352.50** for the desk.

Put into a table the figures calculated above look like this:

Table 11.1   Tracking VAT

Seller	Cost	Tax paid	Sold for	Plus tax collected	Difference paid to Customs and Excise
Estate	–	–	£100	£17.50	£17.50
Furniture maker	£100	£17.50	£150	£26.25	£8.75
Retailer	£150	£26.25	£300	£52.50	£26.25
				Total paid to Customs and Excise	**£52.50**

Notice that each vendor only need pay Customs and Excise the tax collected *less the tax paid*, but all of the net amounts paid add up to the total VAT paid by the final consumer.

Note

If the desk is purchased by a veterinary practice, it will have to pay £300 + £52.50 VAT, but as the practice is VAT registered, once again the VAT can be reclaimed.

However, if the final purchaser is a veterinary nurse who is not VAT registered, then the VAT could not be claimed back and the total net outlay would be £352.50.

Calculation of VAT if the base cost is known

Put simply, the calculation of VAT involves multiplying the base cost by the

$$\frac{\text{VAT rate}}{100}$$

The most common VAT rate is 17.5%. Therefore, to calculate the VAT due on a certain base cost, the latter must be multiplied by

$$\frac{17.5}{100} \quad \text{or} \quad 0.175$$

For instance, the VAT due on a base cost of £120.00

$$= £120.00 \times 0.175 = £21.00$$

Calculating VAT without a calculator

Calculation of VAT can easily be done with the aid of a calculator but there is a simple way to calculate 17.5% of any figure without a calculator. This method is carried out in three easy stages. Notice that 17.5% is made up of 10% + 5% + 2.5%

Therefore by calculating 10% of a figure, which is simply a matter of dividing by 10,

then halving this figure to get 5%,
then halving this figure to get 2.5%,
then adding the three answers gives 17.5%.

Example 1

Calculate 17.5% of £84.40 using the procedure explained above.

10% = £8.44 (divide £84.40 by 10)
5 % = £4.22 (divide the previous answer by 2)
2.5% = £2.11 (divide the previous answer by 2)
Total 17.5% = £14.77 VAT

Check on calculator £84.40 $\times \dfrac{17.5}{100}$ (or £84.40 $\times$ 0.175)

= £14.77
Total price = £84.40 + £14.77 VAT = **£99.17 incl VAT**

Example 2

Calculate 17.5% of £975.23 using the procedure explained above.

10% = £97.523 (divide £975.23 by 10)
5% = £48.7615 (divide the previous answer by 2)
2.5% = £24.38 (divide the previous answer by 2)
Total 17.5% = £170.66 VAT

Check on calculator £975.23 $\times \dfrac{17.5}{100}$ (or £975.23 $\times$ 0.175)

= £170.66
Total price = £975.23 + £170.66 VAT
            = **£1145.89 incl VAT**

Example 3

Calculate 17.5% of £37 .94 using the procedure explained above.

10% = £3.794 (divide £37.94 by 10)
5% = £1.897 (divide the previous answer by 2)

2.5% = £ 0.9485 (divide the previous answer by 2)
Total 17.5% = £ 6.6395 VAT

Check on calculator £37.94 × $\dfrac{17.5}{100}$ (or £37.94 × 0.175)

= £6.6395
= £6.64 (to 2 decimal places)
Total price = £37.94 + £6.64 VAT = **£44.58 incl VAT**

Example 4

Calculate 17.5% of 59p using the procedure explained above.

10% = £0.059 (divide £0.59 by 10)
5% = £0.0295 (divide the previous answer by 2)
2.5% = £0.01475 (divide the previous answer by 2)
Total 17.5% = £0.10325 VAT

Check on calculator £0.59 × $\dfrac{17.5}{100}$ (or £0.59 × 0.175)

= £0.10325
= £0.10 (to 2 decimal places)
Total price = £0.59 + £0.10 VAT = **£0.69 incl VAT**

Example 5

Calculate 17.5% of £1583.91 using the procedure explained above.

10% = £158.391 (divide £1583.91 by 10)
5% = £79.1955 (divide the previous answer by 2)
2.5% = £ 39.59775 (divide the previous answer by 2)
Total 17.5% = £277.18425 VAT

Check on calculator £1583.91 × $\dfrac{17.5}{100}$

(or £1583.91 × 0.175)
= £277.18425
= £ 277.18 (to 2 decimal places)
Total price = £1583.91 + £277.18 VAT
= **£1861.09 incl VAT**

Self-test exercise 1
(fully-worked answers at the end of this chapter)

Calculate the VAT at 17.5% on the following sums of money.

(i)	£23 456.88	(vi)	£177 230.11
(ii)	£10 677.98	(vii)	£89 789.20
(iii)	£1445.96	(viii)	£12 345.59
(iv)	£237.88	(ix)	£17.50
(v)	£53.57	(x)	£2.17

Calculation of VAT from inclusive amounts

VAT is easily calculated on amounts which have no VAT included (see the previous examples). However, the calculation is slightly more complex if the amount given includes VAT and the situation requires that the VAT is split away from the base price. In order to calculate the base price from any VAT inclusive figure, multiply it by:

$$\frac{100}{117.5} \quad \text{or } 0.8510638$$

The amount of VAT can then be found by subtracting the base price from the VAT inclusive figure.

To check if the calculation is correct, the two answers added together should equal the VAT inclusive figure.

Example 1

A bill for servicing an autoclave is £80.00 including VAT. How much did the service cost without VAT? What is the VAT amount?

Calculation

$$\text{Base price} = £80.00 \times \frac{100}{117.5} \text{ (or £80.00} \times 0.8510638)$$
$$= \textbf{£68.09}$$

VAT amount = VAT inclusive figure minus base cost
$$= £80.00 - £68.09$$
$$= \textbf{£11.91}$$
(Amount of bill = £68.09 + £11.91 = £80.00 incl VAT)

Example 2

A new operating table cost £6987.75 including VAT.
How much did the table cost without VAT?
What is the VAT amount?

Calculation

Base price $= £6987.75 \times \dfrac{100}{117.5}$ (or £6987.75 × 0.8510638)

$$= \textbf{£5947.02}$$

VAT amount = VAT inclusive figure minus base cost
$$= £6987.75 - £5947.02$$
$$= \textbf{£1040.73}$$
(Amount of bill = £5947.02 + £1040.73
$$= £6987.75 \text{ incl VAT})$$

Example 3

A box of 12 ballpoint pens costs £2.50 including VAT.
Calculate the base (VAT exclusive) price.

Calculation

Base price $= £2.50 \times \dfrac{100}{117.5}$ (or £2.50 × 0.8510638)

$$= \textbf{£2.13}$$

(Amount of bill = £2.13 + £0.37 = £2.50 (to 2 decimal places) including VAT)

Example 4

An invoice for medical gases is £49.77 including VAT.

Calculate the base (VAT exclusive) price.

Calculation

Base price $= £49.77 \times \dfrac{100}{117.5}$ (or $£49.77 \times 0.8510638$)

$\qquad = \textbf{£42.36}$

(Amount of bill $= £42.36 + £7.41 = £49.77$ (to 2 decimal places) including VAT)

Example 5

A box of 5 laboratory coats costs £135.00 including VAT. Calculate the base (VAT exclusive) price and the amount of VAT paid.

Calculation

Base price $= £135.00 \times \dfrac{100}{117.5}$ (or $£135.00 \times 0.8510638$)

$\qquad = \textbf{£114.89}$

VAT amount $=$ VAT inclusive figure minus base price

$\qquad\qquad = £135.00 - £114.89$

$\qquad\qquad = \textbf{£20.11}$

(Amount of bill $= £114.89 + £20.11 = £135.00$ (to 2 decimal places) including VAT)

Self-test exercise 2
(fully-worked answers at the end of this chapter)

Calculate the **VAT exclusive** amount and **VAT** for each of the following VAT inclusive sums of money:

(i)	£34.56	(ii)	£456.87	(iii)	£231.55
(iv)	£33.57	(v)	£1233.99	(vi)	£531.58
(vii)	£56.97	(viii)	£1237.55	(ix)	£383.77
(x)	£10278.99	(xi)	£864.24	(xii)	£4507.73
(xiii)	£1.55	(xiv)	£0.57	(xv)	£7239.25
(xvi)	£1144.33	(xvii)	£47.92	(xviii)	£23.18
(xix)	£15.57	(xx)	£111.99		

Answers to self-test exercises

Exercise 1

(i) $\dfrac{£23\,456.88}{100} \times 17.5 = £234.5688 \times 17.5 = £4104.95$

(ii) $\dfrac{£10\,677.98}{100} \times 17.5 = £106.7798 \times 17.5 = £1868.65$

(iii) $\dfrac{£1445.96}{100} \times 17.5 = £14.4596 \times 17.5 = £253.04$

(iv) $\dfrac{£237.88}{100} \times 17.5 = £2.3788 \times 17.5 = £41.63$

(v) $\dfrac{£53.57}{100} \times 17.5 = £0.5357 \times 17.5 = £9.37$

(vi) $\dfrac{£177\,230.11}{100} \times 17.5 = £1772.3011 \times 17.5 = £31\,015.27$

(vii) $\dfrac{£89\,789.20}{100} \times 17.5 = £897.8920 \times 17.5 = £15\,713.11$

(viii) $\dfrac{£12\,345.59}{100} \times 17.5 = £123.4559 \times 17.5 = £2160.48$

(ix) $\dfrac{£17.50}{100} \times 17.5 = £0.175 \times 17.5 = £3.06$

(x) $\dfrac{£2.17}{100} \times 17.5 = £0.0217 \times 17.5 = £0.38$

Note

All answers are rounded to two decimal places.

Exercise 2

	Ex VAT	VAT		Ex VAT	VAT
(i)	£29.41	£5.15	(vii)	£48.49	£8.48
(ii)	£388.83	£68.04	(viii)	£1053.23	£184.32
(iii)	£197.06	£34.49	(ix)	£326.61	£57.16
(iv)	£28.57	£5.00	(x)	£8748.08	£1530.91
(v)	£1050.20	£183.79	(xi)	£735.52	£128.72
(vi)	£452.41	£79.17	(xii)	£3836.37	£671.36

(xiii)	£1.32	£0.23	(xvii)	£40.78	£7.14
(xiv)	£0.49	£0.08	(xviii)	£19.73	£3.45
(xv)	£6161.06	£1078.19	(xix)	£13.25	£2.32
(xvi)	£973.90	£170.43	(xx)	£95.31	£16.68

Note

All answers are rounded to two decimal places.

Chapter 12

Examination Techniques

Pre-examination planning

For anyone taking examinations of any kind, it is always a good investment of time to investigate the structure and composition of the examination. Question the lecturers. Look at past papers to see how they are structured.

Veterinary Nursing examinations

Currently, the structure of the Royal College of Veterinary Surgeons (RCVS), Veterinary Nursing examinations consist of two papers, each consisting of 90 multi-choice questions for both Year I and Year II student veterinary nurses (SVNs). Year II have, in addition, four oral and practical sections to the examination, and under the NVQ Scheme these are made up of Laboratory Diagnosis, Radiography, Medical Nursing plus Fluid Therapy, and Surgical Nursing plus Anaesthesia. All questions for both Year I and II students relating to the multi-choice papers, and the oral and practical sections for Year II students, are compulsory.

Throughout the two-year training period, student veterinary nurses also have to complete many specified case log sheets, relating to the patients that they nurse, which are also assessed and verified according to RCVS regulations.

Both Year I and Year II SVNs will be required to carry out calculations which relate to case logs on a day to day basis, and they are often asked to carry out calculations in any one of the different examination sections.

This includes calculations which need to be carried out in a very short time during the practical and oral sections, which can be stressful for many candidates.

However, students are allowed to take basic calculators into both the multi-choice question papers and the orals and practicals. Therefore, provided the basic related mathematical rules have been learnt and application of these has been practised before the examinations, at least some of the stress may be alleviated!

In an examination situation, most mathematical questions will have figures which are reasonably easy to calculate and percentage solutions are likely to have sensible figures to work with. If the answer calculated results in a long convoluted figure, it may be wrong and should be checked, if there is time.

Student veterinary nurses should always make sure when calculating drug doses in a practical and oral examination, that once they have given their answer, they tell the examiner that they would always ask a veterinary surgeon to check the calculation and final drug dosage.

It should not be forgotten, however, that the reason for learning such calculations in the first place is so that this knowledge can be applied by the veterinary nurse on a day to day basis when calculating and administering the various drugs and treatments prescribed by a veterinary surgeon. Although the final dosages given currently remain the legal responsibility of the veterinary surgeon and should be checked by them, quick, accurate calculation and administration of drugs is an important part of most veterinary nurses' duties, often being carried out in a busy and stressful environment.

Administration of a miscalculated dose and subsequent overdose of a drug may cause side effects or in the worst case scenario, cost an animal its life. Conversely, under-dosage could also cause great problems, for example, where an antibiotic under-dose has consequently created a bacterial mutation which is resistant to that particular antibiotic.

Although such events are rare, if veterinary nurses are as skilled as veterinary surgeons at calculating dosages for their patients, miscalculation by either party is more likely to be noticed and rectified long before a drug is administered to a patient.

Examinations in general

For other students from related areas of study who may be using this book as a learning tool, it is essential that they find out from their lecturers and/or the examining body concerned, the answers to such questions as:

How many questions are there?
How many parts to the question are there?
Is there a choice?
Are there any compulsory questions?
How many questions must be answered in total?
Are the questions multi-choice, short answer or essay, or a mixture of these?
What is the duration of the examination?
What aids, if any, can be taken into the examination hall?
Is there an oral and/or practical examination?
Does course work count towards the final marks – if so, what percentage?

All of these questions should be answered early on in a student's course of study.

This preparation will sweep away the 'unknowns' and dispel at least some of the 'myths' surrounding the examination and help to build confidence.

The examination

Many students fail examinations because they don't answer the questions set. Reams of script may be produced, or an answer given in an oral, but this may be what is thought the examiner has asked; or the answer may be slanted towards a vaguely similar subject to that being asked in the question, but with which the student is more familiar.

Whatever the type of question – from multi-choice to essay, before beginning to answer the paper in the examination room, it is worth taking 10 minutes to read the questions carefully.

Try to work out exactly what the examiner is trying to obtain from you. If all questions are compulsory, answer all those which you find easy first. If there is a choice, decide which questions you will be attempting and again, answer the easiest first.

If all questions are compulsory, then attempt all the questions. If a certain amount are required, then attempt that amount. This sounds obvious, but many students leave examinations early with questions left unanswered. Marks can only be awarded for questions answered – some marks may always be gained however little is known about the subject. It is worth trying, especially if there is time to spare.

Questions should not have more time spent on them than is recommended, unless there is time to spare at the end, to 'revisit' questions and improve your answers.

To avoid rushing an answer, work out before starting the apportioned time for each question. Make sure the 10 minutes required to read the paper also figure in the exam question schedule. This way each question will get the time it deserves. Apportion time to each question in relation to the marks awarded, so that a question carrying 20 marks should only be given half the time as one carrying 40 marks.

If possible, also allocate 5 minutes to read through the paper when it is finished. A typical schedule could look like this:

Exam time: 3 hours = 180 min
Reading time: 10 min at start and 5 min at end = 15 min
Questions to be answered in order of attempt:
5, 4, 3, 2, 6 = 5 questions
Marks for the above questions: 10; 30; 20; 10; 30

Start time: 09.00
Read questions until 09.10
Time remaining to answer questions: 165 min (until 11.55)
Reading time at end: 5 min

Timings would have to be approximate, but bearing in mind that the questions allocated the most marks should be allocated the most time, a quickly devised plan for this exam could look like this:

Question	Marks allocated	Time allocated min
		10.0 (read question)
5	10	16.5
4	30	49.5
3	20	33.0
2	10	16.5
6	30	49.5
		5.0 (check answers)
	Total marks 100	Total min 180.0

Most examination bodies expect short, to the point answers, which answer the question exactly (this is the case in both written and oral examinations). Remember, those that set the papers know exactly how long each question should take to answer and appreciate the pressure that students will be under.

Index